VAGUS NERVE

ACTIVATE THE HEALING POWER OF VAGUS NERVE WITH SELF HELP EXERCISES. REDUCE ANXIETY, DEPRESSION, CHRONIC ILLNESS, PTSD, INFLAMMATION, TRAUMA AND MORE

By:

Kevin Kemp

TABLE OF CONTENTS

INTRODUCTION

Imagine it's a Sunday afternoon. You have just had a nice three-course meal and now you sit on the couch to relax and unwind. You feel at peace, so much so that you begin to sleep and fall asleep. While you might think that your body is as comfortable as you are, one of the nervous system divisions is actually hard at work.

The parasympathetic nervous system slows your heart rate, regulates your respiration and calls the organs of your digestive system to order. The time of' rest and digestion' is well underway. One nerve operates tirelessly, this is the Vagus nerve in particular.

The nerve of Vagus is named because it "traverses" like a vagabond and sends sensory fibers to your visceral organs from your brainstem. The Vagus nerve, the largest of the cranial nerves, regulates the parasympathetic nervous system. And it regulates a wide range of key functions, which transmits motor and sensory impulses to each organ in your body. New research has shown that it can also be the missing link to chronic inflammation and the start of an exciting new area of therapy for severe incurable diseases. In this book, the anatomy of the Vagus nerve is studied, including its anatomical course and functions, its medical comparisons.

CHAPTER 1:
THE VAGUS NERVE

Vagus nerve or the tenth cranial nerve (CN X), is mainly associated with the autonomic nervous system's parasympathetic division but also has some sympathetic influence via peripheral chemoreceptors. The Vagus nerve is a mixed nerve, because it has afferent (sensory) as well as efferent (motor) fibers. It ensures that it is not only responsible for carrying motor stimuli to the inner organs, it brings sensory information from these organs back to the central nervous system.

Specifically, Vagus nerve contains:

- General (sensory) fiber afferent
- Special sensory
- Visceral (sensory) fiber afferent
- Branching fiber efferent (motor)
- Visceral fibers efferent (motor).

General afferent fibers are responsible for the sensing from the posterior ear, the external auditory skin, back and outer surface of the tympanic membrane of touch, pain, temperatures and pressure, vibration and proprioceptive sensations. Visceral afferent fibers are responsible for detecting (except pain) the sensory feedback of the viscera or internal organs of the main cavity of the body. Bronchial efferent fibers enclose the muscles, such as mastication muscles, tensor tympani and tensor veli palatini, which develop from the bronchial arches. Special sensory express palate and epiglottis sensation. Visceral fibers, including all smooth muscles and glands, question the viscera.

CRANIAL NERVES

The cranial nerves are 12 pairs of brain nerves that originate mostly in the brainstem. The cranial nerves transmit powerful and afferent signals to and from the body, but primarily to the head and neck. Some of the cranial nerves either produce sensory or motor impulses, while others are mixed and bear the two, like the Vagus nerve. The cranial nerves appear in pairs, but are often described in the singular.

Cranial nerves are also responsible for transmitting sensory signals such as scent, vision, taste, hearing and balance, along with general sensory and motor signals.

WHAT IS VAGUS NERVE?

As previously stated, the body has 12 cranial nerves. They are in pairs and help to link the brain to other parts of the body, like the chest, neck and torso. Others give sensory information to the brain, including information about smells, sights, tastes and sounds. These nerves have sensory functions. Certain cranial nerves control the movement of different muscles and the action of some glans. These are also engine features.

Although some cranial nerves have sensory or motor functions, other nerves have both. The nerve of the Vagus is such a nerve. It is the 10th nerve cranial. It is a functionally diverse nerve that offers many different innervation modalities. The fourth and sixth pharyngeal arches are related. The cranial nerves are numbered according to Roman numerals. Sometimes known as cranial nerve X (CN X), the Vagus nerve.

Vagus nerve is one of many nerves with signals from and to the heart. This helps control internal organs like the heart and abdomen. In the Vagus nerve, nerve fibers are linked to the part of the brain that is believed to cause seizures.

DEVELOPMENT

The central nervous system is said to be in a five vesicle stage by week 6 of pregnancy. The medulla Oblongata comes from myelencephalon. The Vagus nerve motor fibers are produced from the basal plate of medulla Oblongata.

These vesicles are:

- Telencephalon
- Diencephalon
- Mesencephalon
- Metencephalon
- Myelencephalon

The medulla Oblongata comes from myelencephalon. The Vagus nerve motor fibers are produced from the basal plate of medulla Oblongata. In the meantime, the sensory fibers of the vagus nerve come from the cranial neural crest of the ectodermic cell surface.

ORIGIN

There are 4 vagal nuclei in the brainstem's medulla, on which axons of the Vagus nerve emerge or converge.

These include:

- The dorsal motor nucleus
- The Solitary nucleus
- The nucleus ambiguus
- The spinal trigeminal nucleus

The ***Dorsal nucleus*** supplies the parasympathetic efferent mainly to the gastrointestinal system and the pulmonary system are given by the dorsal motor core. The efferent fibers from the ambiguus nucleus supply the pharynx, larynx muscles and soft palate. It also induces branchial efferent fibers and parasympathetic neurons to the brain.

The solitary nucleus receives key afferents and taste information from visceral organs. The afferents converging on the spinal trigeminal nucleus include sensory information about the pain, temperature and depth of the outer ear, the dura of the posterior cranial fossa, and the larynx mucosa.

The Vagus nerve separates the brain from the brain stem medulla oblongata. In addition, the nerves appear between the olive, or the olive skin, and the lower cerebellar peduncle by a series of rootlets. It then passes by the jugular foramen laterally exiting the brain. The sensory ganglia of the Vagus nerve are made of a higher and lower ganglion swelling. The cranial root of the accessory nerve (CN XI) is connected to the Vagus nerve just after this lower ganglion.

In the carotid sheath, the nerve trunk of Vagus then travels down the neck between the carotid artery and the internal jugular vein. The nerve joins the thorax at the base of the neck, yet the Vagus nerve right and left follow different paths after this point. The left Vagus nerve passes before the aortic arch, behind the left main bronchus and into the esophagus. Behind the esophagus and main right bronchus the right Vagus nerve passes.

Through the oesophageal hiatus of the diaphragm the nerves from left to right join the abdomen and take their own separate path to their final branches.

VAGAL NERVE TONE, VARIATION IN HEART RATE AND CHIROPRACTIC

What is vagal tone?

Vagal Tone refers to the level of activity of your vagal nerve. Your Vagal nerve (aka 10th cranial nerve) is a fundamental part of the autonomic nervous system's parasympathetic branch.

This is a deterioration of your nervous system that controls the whole body: healthy people have no less stress in their lives, they are more capable of dealing with stress.

The more the nervous system can deal with life challenges. A healthy person sits mostly in a relaxed state (High Vagal Tone) but has frequent positive pressure variations.

Of example, when you have finished the pressure of a high-intensity exercise is good and your body is mentally happy. The example is the positive feeling after a difficult job has been accomplished. The "I've done it!"Feeling of fulfillment. Will prepare you for the next time, as you think: "I have this!".

Another way has been explained: healthy people have safe communities. What I mean is that the atmosphere frequently switches from rest to constructive stress and relaxation.

Repetitive positive battles or flights are therefore a good thing if the end of the stressful event has a positive emotion. But, "Fight or Flight" long term bouts are not! If you're never able to reach the positive end of the stressful event, it will take you down. For example, everywhere in today's busy life, including work / school stress, financial stress, family and social stress... all of this leads to low-vagal tone, and leads to poor performance and health over a long period.

Is it possible to measure Vagal Tone?

So, how can I know if I spend most of my time stimulating the high vagal nerve?

Most people know intuitively. You either feel stressed, or you experience symptoms that you've learned over time. But it is now easy to measure if you are confused and want to track and chart your progress towards improved vagal nerve stimulation.

In research (in particular Apple Watch), Smart Watches have recently been validated as a reasonably accurate tool for tracking vagal tone variance (HRV).

The Variability of the Heart Rate is the time difference between heartbeats. Oddly enough, it is common to have lapse of time between cardiac beats. The frequency of the beats will however remain constant. Place 2 fingers on your carotid artery, to check yourself; you will find that the beats you exhale are farther apart than when you inhale.

Once you practice, the time lapse is much more consistent between beats.

If you are at rest, you have a high HRV-an indicator of the ability to withstand pressure and, thus, a normal state of strong vagal nerve stimulation (vagal tone)-in time between your heart beats for a few minutes.

If you have a slight difference between heartbeats when at rest, this means that you are on average battling or flying during your day and night and therefore don't have strong vagal tones that lead to poor stress adjustment, and are at risk of poor performance and wellbeing when held for a long time.

In continuous survival mode, which means that you have weak vagal tone (or low heart rate variable), the body is not in an easy state to survive.

Examples of low vagal (or low HRV) symptoms are by age group:

- ***Infant:*** As a baby, you are continually growing! It is therefore important to be in a highly vagal state to facilitate such a climate. Constant crying, knee and hip flexing, frustration, refluxes, poor sleep, poor breastfeeding, poor digestion / bowel movements, poor weight gain are all signs of too much time in the fight or flight mode.

- ***Children:*** Poor sleep, weak development, easily irritated agitation, recurrent colds and ear infections (low immune system) are some examples of their symptoms of low vagal tonus.
- ***Student:*** Depression, poor concentration, poor sleep, poor digestion, constant cold, sometimes exhausted and lack of attention.
- ***Athlete:*** Energy shortages, time to feel calm after run, time to recover, never to recover from injuries, including concussion, power shortage, poor coordination and focus are some examples.
- ***Parent:*** Tired, low concentrations, autoimmune conditions, adrenal fatigue, hypertension, hormonal imbalances are some reasons to lose you composure in children or your spouse.
- ***Grandparent:*** Increased risk of poor health cardiovascular, low energy, grumpiness, dementia.

Where Does Chiropractic Fit in?

Will chiropractic battle all of the above?

No, it does not.

Chiropractic is a physical stress reliever that contributes to a calmer global nervous system (increased vagal tone). It makes you "up," which means that you are more adaptable to stressors in your life.

There are currently several reports on how the Vagus nerve can be activated by drugs and implanted electrodes in the body. It lets the effects transcend what the body does. But the root cause of low Vagus nerve stimulation is not discussed.

FASCINATING FACTS ABOUT THE VAGUS NERVE

Vagus nerve is named because it "wanders" like a vagabond, sending sensory fibers into your visceral organs from your brainstem. The vagus nerve regulates the internal nervous system, the largest of the cranial nerves. And it supervises a wide variety of important functions, which transmit motor and sensory impulses to each organ in your body. New research has shown that the link to chronic inflammation and an exciting new field of treatment for serious, incurable diseases may also be missing. Here are nine facts about this strong nerve bundle.

1. *Vagus Nerve Helps in Preventing Inflammation*

It is okay to have a certain level of inflammation after injury or disease. Yet overabundance is related to many diseases and conditions, rheumatoid arthritis from sepsis to autoimmune. The vagus nerve runs an extensive network of fibers located around all of the organs like spies. This alerts the brain and activates anti-inflammatory neurotransmitters that control the immune response of the body when it is indicated that inflammation is incipient— the production of cytokines or a substance called tumor necrosis factor (TNF).

2. *Helps you in Making Memories*

A research in rats by the University of Virginia found that stimulating the vagus nerves enhanced your memory. The activity released the norepinephrine neurotransmitter into the memory of the amygdala. Related human studies have shown promising treatments for diseases such as Alzheimer's disease.

3. It's Helps You Breath

Acetylcholine, a neurotransmitter produced by a vagus nerve, tells your lungs to breathe. This is why Botox—often used cosmetically—can be potentially dangerous, as it inhibits the development of acetylcholine. However, you can also stimulate the vagus nerve by breathing the abdomen or keeping your breathing for 4-8 counts.

4. It Is Closely Involved With Your Heart

The vagus nerve regulates heart rate by electrical pulsing into the specialized muscle tissue—the heart's internal pacemaker—in the right atrium, where acetylcholine release slows down the pulse. By measuring the time between each heartbeat and then tracking it over time on a charts, doctors can determine your cardiac variability or HRV. Such information can provide insights into heart and vagus nerve resilience.

5. It Enhances Your Body Relaxation Response

The vagus nerve allows the body to relax by releasing acetylcholine as the ever-vigilant and sympathetic nervous system increases fight or flight responses—through the cortisol and adrenaline stress hormone into your skin. The vagus nerve tendrils spread to several species, functioning as fiber-optic cables, and give guidance on the release and remediation of enzymes and proteins such as prolactin, vasopressin and oxytocin. People with a stronger vagus response can recover faster after stress, injury or disease.

6. It Translate Between Your Brain And Your Gut

Your gut uses the vagus' nerve like a walkie's to tell your brain how you feel by electrical impulses known as "action possibilities" your intestines are very real.

7. Overstimulation Of Vagus Nerve Is The Most Crucial Cause Of Fainting

Whether you shudder or are queasy when you see the blood or get a flu shot, you're not weak. The body, due to stress, over-stimulates the vagus nerve, causing blood pressure and heart rate to drop. Blood flow is diverted to your brain during an intense syncope and you lose consciousness. But you have to sit or lie down most of the time to reduce the symptoms.

8. Electrical Of Vagus Nerve Minimizes Inflammation And May Stop It Altogether Stimulation

Neurosurgeon Kevin Tracey has been the first to demonstrate that stimulation to the Vagus nerve can greatly reduce inflammation. Results on rats were so good, the experiment on humans repeated with amazing results. The development of implants in rheumatoid arthritis, which is not regarded as a remedy and is often treated with harmful medications, has shown a drastic decrease and even remission in hemorrhoid and other equally serious inflammatory diseases.

9. Vagus Nerve Stimulation Brought A New Field In Medicine

A new field of medical research, known as bioelectronics, can be the future of medicine, motivated by the positive outcome of vagal nerve stimulation to treat inflammation and epilepsy. With implants that give electrical impulses to different parts of the body, scientists and doctors hope to treat disease with fewer drugs and fewer side effects.

BRANCHES OF VAGUS NERVE

Around the Jugular Fossa

- *Meningeal Branch*

The meningeal branch arises from the upper ganglion and re-enters the skull on the jugular foramen. The meningeal branch re-enters the skull at the jugular foramen. Its section includes general afferent fibers and supplies the dura of the cranial background fossa.

- *Auricular Branch*

The auricular branch, also called Arnold's Nerve, is derived from the superior ganglion and is entered again through the mastoid channel into the lateral portion of the jugular foramen. The branch leaves the tympanomastoid suture of the temporal bone to meet the skin and provide for it. This branch contains all-containing fibers, and it internalizes the external tympanic membrane and provides a small portion of the external ear's back.

Around the Neck

- *Pharyngeal Nerve*

The Pharyngeal nerve Branches of the pharyngeal are derived from the lower nerve ganglion of the Vagus nerve and comprise visceral fibers and motor fibers. The efferent motor fibers are supplied with the pharyngeal nerve attachment (CN XI).

The pharyngeal branch of the Vagus nerve goes through the internal carotid artery into the main pharyngeal muscle. Pharyngeal filaments are formed here by a plexus along with the nervous branches of the Glossopharyngeal (CN IX), the outer laryngeal nerve branches, and the upper cervical ganglion sympathetic fibres. The pharyngeal plexus supplies muscles for the pharyngeal (apart from the muscle of stylopharyngeus), pharyngeal mucosa (apart from the stylopharyngeal muscle), and soft palate (apart from the muscle of the palatin tensor).

Branches of the pharyngeal plexus also contribute with sympathetic and glossopharyngeal fibers to internal plexal carotids (located on the lateral side of the inner carotid artery). The vagal visceral afferent fibers transmit signals from the chemoreceptors in the carotid body.

As the Vagus nerve descends into the carotid sheath, it intercommunicates with filaments or branches of the cervical sympathic spine, which renders it a mixed parasympathic nerve from the neck downward.

- ***Superior laryngeal nerve***

It is the IV-arch structure and thus integrates the derivatives of pharyngeal and laryngeal arch. The afferent fibers of the upper laryngeal nerve come from the lower Vagus nerve ganglion. This section receives some sympathetic cervical ganglion fibers. The upper laryngeal nerve passes between the external and internal carotid arteries at the level crossing of the hypoglossal nerve (CN XII). At the edge of the hyoid bone, under the mandible, it splits into external and internal branches.

The internal laryngeal branch is penetrated by a thyrohyoid membrane into the larynx and contains most of the mucosa above the glottis.

The outer laryngeal branch travels to the lower pharyngeal muscle. The branch is integral to a laryngeal muscle called the muscle of the cricothyroid. The laryngeal nerve, which is another branch of the Vagus nerve mentioned below, intertwines all other intrinsic laryngeal muscles.

- ***Recurrent laryngeal nerves***

There are two recurring laryngeal nerves, one at the right side of the body and one on the left, which are also called lower laryngeal nerves. These are properly called recurrent laryngeal nerves because these follow a recurrent path and go in the opposite direction to the nerve from which they have been branched. The recurrent laryngeal nerve has branchial, ephemeral fibres.

The central nerve trunk is medially attached to the trachea and esophagus and laterally to the common carotid artery, the inner jugular vein and the Vagus nerve. The right nerve branches at the base of the neck from the Vagus nerve, passes under the subclavic artery and then up in the tracheo-esophageal groove and reaches the larynx. The left nerve has a similar path, but it passes around the aortic arch distal to the arteriosus ligament.

The Vagus nerves give off both the right and left recurring laryngeal nerves when they enter the thorax so that they are often included in the thorax branches, especially the right recurrent when they occur in the aortic arch stage. The recurrent nerves then return to the larynx.

As described, the recurrent ipsilateral nerve innerves all the intrinsic laryngeal muscles, apart from cricothyroid muscles. The only exception is the interarytenoid muscle which receives bilateral intervals. The superior and recurrent laryngeal nerves interconnect as ramus contact supplying the esophageal mucosa and smooth muscle with a visceral efferent interview.

- ***Superior cardiac branches***

Superior cardiac nerve branches of the upper (upper) and lower (lower) portions of the neck of the Vagus nerve. Thus, on each side of the upper cardiac nerve are two branches. The upper left branch descends laterally to the trachea, well before the esophagus and to the aortic arch and combines with the deep part of the plexus. The lower left branch also descends laterally to the trachea and then passes the aortic arch and merges with the surface of the heart plexus.

The upper right and lower branches descend deeply into the artery of the sub-clave and diverge into the deep part of the heart plexus.

Around the Thorax

- ***Inferior cardiac nerve***

The lower cardiac nerve on the left side is a consequence of the recurrence of the laryngeal nerve. On the right side, it comes from the Vagus trunk next to the trachea. In the inner part of the cardiac plexus both left and right branches end.

The cardiac plexus, which is responsible for the innervation of the heart, receives fibers from the Vagus cardiac nerves and from recurrent laryngeal nerves.

- ***Anterior Bronchial branches***

On the anterior surface of the lung root are found two or three small, anterior bronchial branches. Such roots, together with contributions from the sympathetic trunk, form the anterior plexus which surrounds the bronchial tree and the visceral pleura.

- ***Posterior bronchial branches***

They are generally larger and more frequent than the middle branches and are situated on the rear root of the lung. Such branches form the rear pulmonary plexus together with contributions from the sympathetic trunk's third and fourth ganglia. The pulmonary plexus behind intersects the same structures as its ancestor.

- ***Esophageal branches***

The esophagus plexus consists of esophageal branches of the Vagus nerve together with visceral branches of the sympathetic trunk. The esophagus branches extend to the bronchial plexus from above and below.

Oesophageal plexus filaments on the back side of the pericardium. The esophagus is motor and sensory to the esophagus.

<u>Around the Abdomen</u>

- *Gastric branches*

These are the branches of the right Vagus nerve forms the back gastric plexus at the postero-lower surface of the stomach, while the left Vagus nerve branches form anterior gastric plexus on the anterior upper surface of the abdomen. All distinctions operate between the less complex surfaces.

In addition to posterior gastric branches, the anterior gastric fibers spread to the upper part of duodenum and the pylorus, while posterior vagal trunk sends fibers to major, autonomous abdominal plexuses from which vagal fibers are dispersed over the areas of the celiac, renal and superior mesenteric arteries.

- ***Celiac branches***

The celiac branches of the Vagus nerve are derived mainly from the right vagus nerve. Such divisions are connected with the celiac plexus that is inside the pancreas, lungs, spleen, supra-arenal bodies and intestines.

- ***Hepatic branches***

Hepatic branches The Vagus nerve hepatic branches are derived mainly from the Vagus nerve left. Both branches enter the liver plexus inside the liver.

OVERVIEW

- ***Sensory:*** Innerves in the skin of external acoustic meat and the laryngopharynx and larynx internal surfaces. Provides heart and abdominal tactile feeling.
- ***Special sensory:*** supplies the epiglottis and tongue root with the taste sensation.
- Parasympathetic: Innervates the trachea, bronchi, and gastrointestinal tract, and controls the heart rhythm.
- ***Motor:*** Provides motor innervation to most pharynx, soft palate and larynx muscles.

The functions can be divided into seven classes even further. One is to regulate the nervous system.

However, there are two main parts of the nervous system: sympathetic and parasympathetic. The friendly side increases attention, strength, blood pressure, heart rate and breathing rate.

The parasympathetic side of the Vagus nerve reduces anxiety, blood pressure and heart rate, and it helps calm, relaxation and digestion. Due to this, Vagus nerve as well helps in urination, sexual arousal and defecation.

Other Vagus nerve benefits include the following:

- ***Interaction between the brain and the intestine:*** The Vagus nerve provides information from the intestine to the brain.
- ***Deep-breathing relaxation:*** the nerve of Vagus interacts with the diaphragm. A person feels more relaxed with deep breaths.
- ***Reduction of inflammation:*** The Vagus nerve sends a signal of anti-inflammation to the rest of the body.
- ***Increasing cardiac velocity and blood pressure:*** If the Vagus nerve becomes

overactive, it may result in the heart not pumping out enough blood around the body. Excessive nerve activity of the Vagus may in some cases cause loss of consciousness and organ damage.

- ***Anxiety management:*** The Vagus nerve sends information from the intestine to your brain linked to the managing of stress, anxiety and fear, which is why it says "good feeling."

- **SPECIAL SENSORY EFFECTS**

The Vagus nerve has a littler role in perception of the taste. It has afferent fibers from the tongue and epiglottis root.

(This should not be confused with the particular sensation of the glossopharyngeal nerve that gives the retro 1/3 of the tongue the taste sensation).

- **MOTOR EFFECTS**

The Vagus nerve cycles most of the pharynx and larynx muscles. Both muscles are responsible for swallowing and phonation initiation.

Pharynx

Some pharyngeal muscles are interspersed with the pharyngeal branches of a vaginal nerve:

- Palato-pharyngeus
- Salpingo-pharyngeus
- Superior, middle and inferior pharyngeal muscles

Larynx

Innervation is done through the recurrent laryngeal nerve and outer branch of the upper laryngeal nerve.

Laryngeal nerve:

- Lateral crico-arytenoids
- Vocalis
- Tranverse and oblique arytenoids
- Posterior crico-arytenoid
- Thyro-arytenoid

External Laryngeal nerve:

- Cricothyroid

Other Muscles

Including larynx and pharynx, the Vagus nerve also internalizes the palatoglossus of the laryngeal and the rest in the soft palate muscles.

- PARASYMPATHETIC EFFECT

In the abdomen and thorax, the Vagus nerve is the primary parasympathetic connection to the heart and gastrointestinal organs in the thorax and abdomen.

The Heart

Cardiac branches begin in the thorax and send parasympathetic intervals to the sino-atrial or atrio-ventricular nodes of the heart (See here for more cardiac anatomy).

Both divisions promote a decrease of the rest of the heart rate. They are always involved and produce 60 to 80 beats per minute tempo. If the Vagus nerve is damaged, the rest heart rate is about 100 beats per minute.

Gastro-intestinal system

The Vagus nerve provides most abdominal organs with parasympathetic innervation. It serves branches to the esophagus, stomach and most intestinal tract—up to the massive colon splenic bending.

The Vagus nerve's function is to stimulate smooth muscle and glandular secretions in these bodies. In the stomach, for example, the Vagus nerve increases gastric emptying levels and improves the production of acid.

CLINICAL SIGNIFICANCE: DISORDERS OF THE VAGUS NERVE

Cardiovascular

Many pharmacological agents can be used to enable cardiovascular tone to slow down the cardiac rate. Beta-blockers, muscarinic agonists and cardiac glycosides, including Digoxin, may only be used.

During an emotional stress phase, for instance, a vasovagal syncope may result in a sudden drop in the blood pressure and heart rate. In addition, a carotid massage can compress the carotid sinus which results in a high blood pressure perception. This will result in CN X rising firing, leading to lower SA node and AV node operation. Generally there will be a reduced frequency and intensity of contraction and syncope.

Some congenital heart defects, like the patent ductus arteriosus, can irritate the larynx nerve of the left recurrent nerve and contribute to dysphony.

Gastro-intestinal

CN X lesions are rare. A pharyngeal branch injury can lead to dysphagia (difficulty swallowing) due to involvement in the pharynx muscles. As CN X separates the muscles Palatopharyngeus and Salpingopharyngeus, an injury may result in the palatoglossary arch falling away from Uvula. The CN IX is sensory to the oropharynx and to the laryngopharynx, with CN X as the engine efferents of the Gag reflex, hence a loss of the Gag reflex in this region.

A vagotomy could once be done to reduce the production of excess stomach acid. Nevertheless, this is no longer necessary with developments in pharmacology therapy.

Other

As mentioned above a lesion causes dysphonia to one of the RLNs. An injury to both the RLN can cause aphonia and a stridor (inspiratory wheeze). RLN paralysis is usually caused by larynx or thyroid cancer or operating complications.

CHAPTER 2:
WHAT HAPPENS WHEN VAGUS NERVE DOES NOT WORK?

A small investigation of the Vagus nerve finds a whole host of conditions that are either related positively or are currently being examined for a connection with the nerve. Which vary from mild frustration to major problems. If you are affected by a continuum everywhere, it can of course affect your overall feeling of well-being and results.

Many people will experience a vasovagal reaction at some stage because of pressure or over-stimulation. Blood pressure decreases, the heart rate decreases, and the blood vessels in your legs widen, which can cause nausea or decay. This is normally a mild reaction, but some people who experience it more frequently may have to seek medical help.

Many problems associated with Vagus dysfunction include: obesity, depression, mood disorders, bradycardia, gastrointestinal diseases, chronic inflammation, fainting and convulsion.

Of course, most of these conditions can lead to further diseases, such as obesity and inflammation, both associated with cancer as well as diabetes. Anxiety or mood disorders can also cause depression.

Nerve Damage

Vagus nerve damage can have a variety of symptoms because the nerve is so long and affects multiple areas.

Potential symptoms of damage to the nerve includes:

- Loss of voice or difficulty speaking
- A voice that is wheezy or hoarse
- Problem drinking liquids
- Pain in the ear
- Loss of the gag reflex
- Abnormal heart rate
- Abnormal blood pressure
- Vomiting or Nausea
- Lower production of stomach acid
- Abdominal bloating or pain

Someone's symptoms may depend on which part of the nerve.

Gastroparesis

Professionals believe that a condition called gastroparesis could also be caused by damage to the Vagus nerve. This typical condition affects the involuntary contractions of the digestive system, preventing proper emptying of the stomach.

Symptoms of gastroparesis include:

- Nausea or vomit, especially vomiting of untaxed foods after eat
- Loss of appetite or fullness shortly after meal begins
- Reflux of acid
- Abdominal pain or bloating
- Unexplained weight loss
- Blood sugar fluctuations

Many patients develop gastroparesis following a vagotomy operation that eliminates all or part of the vagus nerve.

Risk Factors

There are so many factors that can increase your risk of Gastroparesis, and these factors include the following:

- Diabetes
- Abdominal or esophageal surgery
- Infection, commonly the virus
- Other medicines that slow the rate of emptying of the abdomen, such as drugs for pain
- Scleroderma
- Nervous system disorders such as Parkinson's disease or multiple sclerosis
- Hypothyroidism (low thyroid) Females are m

NOTE: Women are most likely to have Gastroparesis than men

Complications

Gastroparesis can cause many complications, such as:

- *Acute dehydration* can be caused by persistent vomiting.
- *Malnourishment.* Low appetite will prevent you from consuming enough calories or from eating enough nutrients because of vomiting.

- ***Food that will harden and remains in the belly***. Undigested food will harden into a solid mass called a bezoar in your stomach. Bezoar can cause nausea and vomiting and can be life-threatening if food does not reach your small intestine.

- ***Unpredictable fluctuations in blood sugar***. While gastroparesis causes no diabetes, frequent changes in the rate and amount of food in the small bowel may result in erratic changes in blood sugar levels. These fluctuations in blood sugar worsen diabetes. In effect, inadequate blood sugar control exacerbates gastroparesis.

- ***Reduced quality of life***. The acute worsening of the symptoms can make working and other tasks challenging.

Vasovagal Syncope

The Vagus nerve often overreacts to some stress factors, for instance:

- Extreme heat exposure
- Bodily harm
- Vision of the blood or drawing of blood

- Discomfort, like bowel movements
- Standing for a long time.

Note, the Vagus nerve activates certain cardiovascular muscles which help slow heart rate. If it overreacts, the heart rate and blood pressure can suddenly fall and become weak. This is called a vasovagal syncope.

Emotional and Physical Effects

Excessive stimulation of the vagal nerve during emotional stress, which is a parasympathetic overcompensation for a powerful sympathetic stress-associated nervous system response, could also trigger vasovagal syncope due to an unexpected decrease in cardiac output, resulting in cerebral hypo-perfusion. Vasovagal syncope more than other classes affects young children and women. It may also lead to temporary bladder control loss under extreme fear moments.

Evidence has shown that women with full spinal cord injuries will experience Vagus nerve orgasms from the uterus and cervix to their brains.

Insulin signaling activates the potassium (KATP) sensitive channels of adenosine triphosphate (ATP) in the arcuate nucleus, reduces Agouti-Related Protein release (AgRP), and, through Vagus nerve, reduces liver glucose production by the reduction of glucose enzymes: Phosphoenolpyruvate carboxykinase, Glucose6-phosphatase.

Vagus Nerve and Anxiety

The sympathetic nervous system is triggered when we are exposed to stressful situations. If the stress continues and the physiological response which it causes can not be switched off. it will not take long before problems appear. It includes the activation on the brain level of two pathways: the hypothalamic-hypophysical-adrenal axis and the brain-intestinal axis.

Through raising hormone (CRF) output from the hypothalamus to the hypophysis, the brain responds to pressure and anxiety and stimulates another hormone (ACTH), which in effect passes through the bloodstream to the surrenal glans, stimulating the cortisol and adrenaline secretion, as immune suppressers and inflammatory precursors.

Anxiety and chronic stress cause an increase in the brain's glutamate, a neurotransmitter that causes migraines, depression and anxiety when generated in excess. In addition, a high cortisol level reduces hippocampus volume, the part of the brain that creates new memories.

The Vagus nerve involvement contributes to symptoms including dizziness, gastrointestinal disorders, pacing, respiratory difficulties and disproportionate emotional response. Indeed, the sympathetic nervous system keeps the Vagus nerve active as it is impossible to activate the relaxation signal, causing the person to react impulsively and suffer of anxiety.

It is also interesting that a study at Miami University found that the vagal tone was passed from mother to child. Women with anxiety, depression or great rage during pregnancy also had less vagal activity and lower levels of dopamine and lower vagal activity and serotonin in their children.

Vagus Nerve Testing

The doctor may examine the gag reflex to test the Vagus nerve. Doctor can use a soft cotton swab to tickle the back of the throat on both sides during this part of the examination. This should make the person fuck. If the person doesn't cough, this may be because of a Vagus nerve problem.

WAYS TO REACTIVATE YOUR VAGUS NERVE

Here are my five ways to reactivate your distinctly vagus nerve:

1. Re-establish the vagus nerve

Every morning I sat on my chair, drank a few snacks of coffee, and began phase 1 — clearing my vacuum nerve with the following sequence to help loosen and relieve pressure.

-        Place your right index and middle finger over your navel and push it to the right and inside.

- Take the same two fingers and press over your navel, then to the left again. Then press right, center and left (about one inch above the navel).

- On the other side, force the 3 finger pads into your skin at top of the head (on the back), then move the fingers into the middle of your skirt (on the chest) and on the front (on the front).

- Do the procedure at the same time by putting a hand right above the navel and squeezing the head of the other hand. Repeat three times, at the end put your arms down, close your eyes and breathe. You will feel your breath getting deeper, the loosening of your mouth, the loosening of your neck and the shifting away of your eyes. Try again if you don't hear something.

2. *Fear tap*

The "fear tap" technique calms the fight or the flight response, eliminates irrational fear and protects the mind. First, flip one hand over so that the palm looks down. Take your fingers and place them halfway between your wrist and hand, between your ring finger and pinky finger, on the back of your hand. Tap this region for 30 to 60 seconds, breathe in through your nose and out in your mouth with two or three fingers.

3. *Cow / cat stretch*

The stretch of cat / cow I often do. This is a yoga asana that is one of the best ways to boost the vagus nerve. Here's a version sitting. Sit down with your feet on the edge of a chair about the width of the knee. Put your hands on your thighs, and as you exhale, tuck your chin in to the thigh around your back, just like a frightened cat. Then inhale, open your back, and draw your heart forward as you return your shoulder blades. Inhale and exhale (squeeze out your heart, round up). Enable your breathing to make your spine more flexible.

4. *Hands to Forehead*

Another way to reduce reactivity is by vigorously rubbing your hands together about 10 seconds before putting a hand on your forehead and the other on your forehead. It looks like you are testing for a fever in your head. You pull the blood up to the forebrain by putting your hands into this position, closing your eyes for 20 seconds, and breathing into the lower belly. As this occurs, reactivity decreases. You will be aware of this because when you take away your hands (place them palm down on your lap), your breath comes from your lower abdomen.

5. *Body scan*

Once you recognize your reactivity level, scan the entire body again quickly. Keep your eyes closed or softly open, start at the top and move your feet to the bottom. Scanning your body is like getting your oven preheated. Your oven needs to be a certain temperature to adequately cook your food inside and outside, so that your body can absorb your emotions in some way–i.e., free of reactivity.

Clearing reactivity in the morning is best done because your body digests the stressors of the day when you sleep. Taking the following test 10 seconds out of your morning:

-       Sit down or stand up with your arms parallel to the floor, and your feet.

-       Inhale.

-       Using your mind, trace your feet slowly from the top of your head to the soles (on the exhale).

Digestion and the Vagus Nerve

Digestion is out of whack when vagus function is extinguished. Symptoms may include heart burn or GERD, IBD, or inflammatory bowel diseases such as ulcerative colitis, which can prevent a body from healing the common cause of Irritable Bowel Syndrome (IBS) Small Intestine Bacterial Overgrowth (SIBO).

Vagus nerve is part of the system that tells the stomach to expel digestive acids and juices and start the intestinal movement. When we chew our food, we begin to mix the fibers in our food with the digestive acids and enzymes that break down food before it reaches our stomach before it flows into the large and small intestines.

If the vagus nerve does not get or give the right signals, the food-mixed-acid stream through the intestines slows down. This means that bacterial, yeast or parasite overgrowths— as well as used hormones and toxins the body worked to remove from the body — slowly move through the intestines. The risk of IBS and SIBO is increased with increased exposure to bacteria, waste products, and potentially worsening infections. More hormones than your body planned can lead to hormones being exposed to balance.

CHAPTER 3:
CAUSES OF VAGUS NERVE DAMAGE

- **Diabetes**

Diabetes can lead to neuropathy or damage to the nerves in a variety of parts of the body. A long increase in diabetes blood sugar can alter nerve chemistry and damage the nerve supporting blood vessels.

For cases where diabetes has weakened the Vagus, gastroparesis can occur, a disorder in which the intestine and stomach muscles cannot effectively transfer food through the gastrointestinal system. In symptoms such as nausea, diarrhea, heartburn, constipation, bowel bloat, spasm and decreased appetite, gastroparesis exists.

- **Alcoholism**

Chronic alcohol abuse, known as alcoholic neuropathy, causes nerve damage. The abuse of alcohol impacts the autonomic nervous system with a dose-related toxic effect, which involves the Vagus nerve. Abstaining from alcohol will reverse the Vagus nerve damage.

- **Infection and surgical complications**

Following upper respiratory viral infections, vagus nerve damage can occur. Typically, signs of these diseases include cough, nasal congestion and runny nose. Symptoms that continued with cough, throat clearing, speech disturbances and vocal exhaustion in the patients described as posterior vagal neuropathy or PVVN.

The Vagus nerve may be damaged during stomach or small intestine surgery. A procedure called laparoscopic hemic fundoplication was associated with damage to the vagus nerve.

VAGUS NERVE IN MEDICAL THERAPY

Because of the many important functions of the vagus nerve, medical science has been involved for decades with the concept of the medical therapy with the aid of vagus nerve stimulation or vagus nerve blockage.

The vagotomy procedure (cutting the nerve of Vagus) was a key element of treatment of peptic ulcer disease for decades as it reduced the level of peptic acid produced by the stomach. The vagotomy however had some negative effects and is now much less commonly used with the advent of more effective treatment.

Today, the use of electronic stimulators (mainly altered pacemakers) to continuously stimulate the vagus nerve to treat various medical conditions is of great interest. These devices (generally referred to as Vagus nerve stimulants, or VNS devices) have been widely used in the treatment of people with severe epilepsy that is drug-refractory. VNS therapy is also used to treat refractory anxiety occasionally.

As everything looks like a nail when you have a hammer, companies that produce VNS devices examine their use in several other conditions, including high blood pressure, migraines, tinnitus, fibromyalgia and weight loss.

In addition, these VNS applications are promising. Nevertheless, once the hysteria is replaced by solid clinical evidence, the true potential of VNS will emerge.

MEDICAL METHODS AND TREATMENTS FOR VAGUS NERVE

Vagus Nerve Stimulation

A growing body of research suggests we can control or hack the Vagus nervous system. Vagus hacks date from work by Kevin Tracey in 1998. Through his research, he discovered that he can reduce the body's inflammatory response by stimulating the Vagus nerve with an electrical impulsion.

This has positive consequences for the treatment of conditions such as Crohn's disease, rheumatism and other inflammatory diseases. The work of Tracey is the basis of the concept of bioelectronics to treat disorders such as anxiety and epilepsy are now used.

In addition to these conditions, inflammation is a response, often caused by stress that we all have in our bodies. For some, anxiety and inflammatory response can be persistent, leading to other health problems.

Vagus nerve stimulation involves placing an instrument that simulates the nerve using electrical impulses in the body. It is used to treat such epilepsy and depression cases that do not respond to other therapies.

Typically the unit is placed under the chest skin, where the wire attaches it to the left nerve of the vagus. Once the device is activated, the device sends signals to your brain stem through the vagus nerve and then sends information to your brain. The unit is normally controlled by a neurologist, but often a portable magnet is used by individuals to power the device.

Vagus nerve stimulation is thought to help combat a variety of other disorders in the future, including multiple sclerosis, Alzheimer's disease and headaches of the clusters.

Vagus nerve stimulation is a procedure used to minimize seizure frequency and intensity if medication is not successful.

This involves placing a small electric stimulator on the neck around the nerve of the Vagus and a power source close to the axis or heart. The system acts like a heart pacemaker to activate the left nerve of Vagus. It sends intermittent electric signals to the brain automatically and can be triggered manually to avoid a beginning seizure.

Clinical trials have tested the efficacy of Vagus nerve stimulation. Accordingly, two separate conditions have been approved for use by the United States Food and Drug Administration (FDA).

Epilepsy

The FDA approved the use of Vagus nerve stimulation for refractory epilepsy in 1997.

It involves a small electrical tool that is in a person's chest, similar to a pacemaker. A thin wire known as a lead flows to the Vagus nerve from the system.

The system is put under general anesthesia in the body by surgery. It then transmits the electric impulses to the brain via the vagus nerve at regular intervals, throughout the day, to minimize or even avoid seizures.

Side effects of the Vagus nerve stimulation include:

- Sort throat
- Change in voice

- Coughing
- Shortness of breath
- Difficulty swallowing
- Nausea or stomach discomfort

Patients who use the drug should always inform their physician if they have any concern as there may be ways to reduce or avoid epilepsy.

Who Can Benefit From This Stimulation

Patients whose seizures are not controlled by medication and who lose consciousness during complex partial seizures or general seizures, may benefit from vagal nerve boost.

Such medication will lead to less or less serious convulsions, although not everyone can see a difference. In all cases, the patient needs to continue taking anti-epileptic medications before inserting the stimulator. In some cases, the neurologist may recommend a reduction in medication some months after the implantation of a vagal nerve stimulator.

Evaluation

A doctor will typically have to thoroughly assess the patient's medical condition before inserting a vagal nerve stimulator. You have to go through the medical record, inquire about the medical history of the patient and the immediate medical history of the family. Data on any medications the patient may have taken, including electronic drugs, vitamins, nutritional supplements and herbal remedies should be registered. All medicines are accessible.

Procedure

During an operation that takes one to two hours, the vagal nerve stimulator is implanted. The stimulator is attached to a nerve in the neck by a wire. The stimulator is scheduled to periodically activate the nerve. The stimulator battery must be replaced roughly every 10 years. This can be achieved with local anesthesia during a simple procedure that does not require a hospital stay.

The patient may have some tingling or hoarseness in the neck during the pulsation. With time, many people get used to these feelings.

The doctors are taking care to ensure that the vagal nerve stimulator functions properly and helps control seizures of the patient.

The benefits of VNS may be:

- Having less severe seizures
- Having fewer seizures
- Having enhanced quality of life
- Possibly less epilepsy medication

You can find that your emergency management is improving slowly over time. Six out of ten people with VNS fit consider that their number is halved. Nonetheless, problems suit between three and six in a hundred people with VNS. These were generally associated with disease and sorted by a second operation.

SOME FREQUENTLY ASKED QUESTIONS ABOUT VAGUS NERVE STIMULATION

Can I have VNS Therapy?

Many national health policy authorities have recommendations on who should VNS be given or not. National Health Service (NHS) in the UK, for instance, has recommendations which only people with epilepsy may have. It is limited when other therapies have not succeeded or are not suitable, to adults and children with epilepsy. To be considered for VNS treatment, although you have taken a variety of epileptic drugs, you still have seizures, or the epileptics give you too many side effects. You also need to be uncomfortable for brain epilepsy operation, or you have had brain operation but still have seizures.

What is involved with VNS surgery?

A neurosurgeon performs surgery to implant the VNS system, usually with general anesthesia. The treatment takes 1 to 2 hours, and usually the same day or the next day you go home. The neurosurgeon makes two small cuts, one in a pin to the left of your neck and the other on the left of your head, under your collarbone. The generator is mounted in your chest under the body. A lead is put under the skin to connect the generator in the neck to the left vagus nerve. As with any method, there is a small risk of anesthetic reaction. The risk of infection and bleeding is also low. Before the procedure, your surgeon will send you more details.

Following VNS surgery, you might have some discomfort from the implant region for a while. There's something the doctor can prescribe for this.

What's happen after VNS operation?

Typically, the generator is switched off for two weeks after the service. This allows the body to recover. After that, a specialist nurse in a hospital usually turns it on. We will through the settings slowly over a few weeks. It gives you an opportunity over time to get used to stimuli.

Do I still need to take epilepsy medication after the VNS is fitted?

VNS was intended to be used, not to replace it, in addition to epilepsy medication. Many people need to continue to take epilepsy after a VNS system has been installed. Some people may reduce the amount of epilepsy medication they take. You should discuss any possible changes to your medication with your epilepsy specialist.

How long does this last?

The generator will have to be replaced at some stage if the battery is low. Depending on the model and the settings used, the battery can last for between 3 and 8 years. A doctor or nurse will inform you when the battery fails during your follow-up. They will then plan the installation of a new generator. It requires a small operation that lasts less than an hour.

How do I get a replacement magnet?

Tell your epilepsy specialist nurse if you need a replacement magnet. You should be able to supply a new magnet for free.

Why Should I Be Careful If I Have VNS?

- ***MRI scans***

In case you are recommended to have an MRI, it is critical that all participants know the VNS system. You may need to take precautions to safely perform the scan. You should have a neurologist patient MRI form to show people who are doing the MRI scan.

- ***Airport security scanners***

Safety scanners of the airport should not impact or harm the system. VNS Therapy device manufacturers recommend that you provide the airport security with your VNS Therapy ID card in order to be safe. Instead, you may order a pat-down search.

Certain devices that know that they are close other types of equipment will affect your generator.

- The doctor will tell you if it is safe for you to be where pacemaker warning signs are. Since equipment that might affect a pace manufacturer may also affect your VNS generator
- Stay at least 60 cent or 2 feet away from shop deactivators of Electronic Article Surveillance

System labels. This will prevent your generator from being triggered. The deactivators can usually be found in shop entrances.

- Tablets and their cover, haircuts, vibrators and laundries can all be equipped with electromagnetic fields which you must keep at least 20 cm or 8 inches away from your chest. If your generator is switched on, just move away from the system that causes the problem.

VAGOTOMY

Vagotomy is an essential component of peptic (duodenal and gastric) ulcer (PUD) surgery.

Vagotomy is a type of operation that eliminates all or part of the nerve of the Vagus. Although vagotomy procedures were standard treatment for stomach ulcers, medication advances and a better understanding of the bacteria in the intestine have made them less frequent. These are usually performed in combination with other treatments, such as pyloroplastic.

Why is that done?

Vagotomies are commonly used to treat peptic ulcers by reducing the amount of acid released by the stomach. It's rarely done on its own these days. Then, people usually begin to take antibiotics to kill an H. Inhibitors of pylori infection or proton pump to suppress stomach acid.

When medicines alone are not effective, doctors suggest a vagotomy operation in conjunction with:

- ***Resection.*** This is done to remove a damaged or ill digestive tract component.

- ***Abdominal drainage***. It extracts extra abdominal fat, known as ascites.\

- ***Pyloroplastic.*** This operation enlarges the pylorus near the end of the abdomen. This helps to control the movement in the small intestine of partially digested food and digestive juices.

- ***Diversion.*** The gastrointestinal (GI) tube is adapted to pass around the injured or diseased portion of the digestion process.

However, research suggests that they can help also to treat:

- Obesity
- Diabetes
- Pulmonary fibrosis

SPECIFIC VAGOTOMY FOR VARIOUS PURPOSES

- ***Truncal vagotomy.*** Many forms of vagotomy are used. This is commonly used for pyloroplasty or abdominal drainage in the treatment of chronic peptic ulcers. This includes the cutting off one or more branches that divide the main trunk of the Vagus nerve into the stomach and other digestive organs through the esophagus.

- ***Selective vagotomy.*** Another choice cuts down the vagus nerve closer to the organs to eliminate only some of its work. It is a good choice to treat stomach ulcers without having a major effect on other organs, such as the liver, that are based on the Vagus nerve.

- ***Highly selective vagotomy.*** This form of vagotomy involves only removing the part of the Vagus nerve that affects the stomach directly, retaining many of the other functions of the Vagus nerve. This form is usually accompanied by truncal vagotomy.

Patient will be under general anesthesia for each type.

How is recovery?

After a vagotomy operation, the patient will typically have to spend for one week in the hospital. Drain extra stomach acid regularly when observing the patient's body reaction to the treatment.

Following about one week, the doctor must remove the stitches unless they are removed.

It takes approximately six weeks to recover fully. The physician can recommend following a liquid diet until the GI tract adapts to the changes in Vagus nerve function.

The person will probably avoid as much as possible acidic or spicy foods.

Are there any risk involved?

Vagotomy surgeries carry the same potential risks as many other types of operations, including:

- Internal bleeding
- Shock from blood loss
- Infections
- Trouble urinating
- Deep vein thrombosis
- Allergic anesthesia reactions

Patient also carries a risk of dumping syndrome. This enables food to move through the stomach rapidly without being digested properly. Such effects can occur immediately after treatment, and become less severe when a digestive system improves. The symptoms include:

- Rapid heartbeat after eating
- Abdominal cramps
- Diarrhea
- Nausea and vomiting

The Vagus nerve does not have to be shocked. Compared to a muscle, it can be toned and reinforced. Listed below are some basic things you can do that will greatly improve your health:

1. ***Social Relationships.*** A research allowed participants to think compassionately about others and secretly echo optimistic words about friends and family. Positive social relationships. Compared with the monitors, the meditators displayed an overall increase in positive feelings after the session, such as serenity, pleasure and hope. Such positive thoughts of others contributed to an increase in slightly functional variability of the heart rate. The results showed a Vagus nerve more toned than when meditating.

2. ***Cold*** – "Cold exposure like cold shower or facial dunking also stimulates the nerve," says Mentore.

   Studies show that the fight or flight process decreases and the rest and digester (parasympathetic) mechanism increases as the body adapts to the cold, and this is regulated by the vagus nerve. Some form of acute cold exposure like drinking cold ice water may increase activation of the Vagus nerve.

3. ***Gargling*** - Another home remedy is to gargle with water for an under-stimulated vagus nerve. In fact, gargling stimulates the pallet muscles that are fired by the Vagus nerve.

"Usually, patients are going to tear a little and, if they don't, we advise that they do so periodically before they find that they start to tear up a little," says Hoffman. "It has been shown that this increases memory performance instantly." So first gargle it before you drink water.

4. ***Singing and singing*** - Humming, song singing, hymn singing, and upbeat enthusiastic singing all increase the variability in the heart rate (HRV). Singing is basically like starting a vagal pump which sends calming waves. Also, singing at the top of your lungs works to activate the vagus with muscles in the back of the throat. Powerful singing stimulates both the

sympathetic nervous system and the vagus nerve which helps to flow. Singing in unison, frequently performed in churches and synagogues, often improves the work of HRV and Vagus. It has been found that singing increases oxytocin and is also known as the love hormone because it helps people to feel closer.

Compassion was shown to contribute to a stronger Vagus nerve.

5.   *Massage -* You can stimulate the vagus nerve by massaging your feet and neck through the carotid sinus on both sides of the body. A neck massage can contribute to reducing convulsions. A foot massage will reduce the cardiovascular and blood pressure. Vagus nerve can as wel be stimulated by a pressurized massage. Such massages help infants gain weight by improving intestinal activity, primarily by activating the vagus nerve.

6.   *Laughter* – "Laughter is the best medicine," as the saying suggests. Most studies show laughter's health benefits. Bliss and happiness

are normal promoters of resistant. Laughter also activates the nerve of the Vagus. Research shows that laughter in a group environment improves HRV (heart rate variation).

There are many cases where people are fainting because of laughter and this can be caused too much by the vagus nerve / parasympathetic system. Fainting and urination, vomiting, swallowing or bowel movements may accompany the laugh–all of which are accompanied by activation of the vagus. A good laugh is good for cognitive function and protects from heart disease. It also improves beta-endorphins and nitric oxide, and the vascular system gains

7. ***Yoga & Tai Chi*** - Both increase the function of the vagus nerve and the parasympathic system in general. Studies have demonstrated that yoga increases GABA, a soothing brain neurotransmitter. Researchers think this is achieved by "stimulating vagal afferents (fibers)," which increase parasympathetic

nervous system function. This is especially helpful for people coping with anxiety or depression.

Studies show that tai chi can also "boost vagal synchronization." 8. Breathing Deeply And Slowly–Breathing techniques came into the west around the 70's, but East practitioners used these approaches for thousands of years. There is a solid science behind deep breathing–both can activate the vagus nerve and increase the HRV.

The heart and neck have neurons called baroreceptors that sense blood pressure and transmit the neuronal signal to the brain. The vagus nerve which links the heart to less blood pressure and a lower heart rate is activated. Slow respiration, with approximately equal breathing periods, improves baroreceptor sensitivity and vagal activation. It can be beneficial to breathe between 5-6 breaths per minute in the average adult.

8.   ***Deep breathing*** is now widely accepted to play a key role in maintaining a healthy physiological balance. In a 2014 paper, Lehrer and Gevirtz are discussing a wide range of interesting explanations why HRV biofeedback works, reiterating that diaphragmic respiration is part of a feedback loop that enhances the vagal toning by enhancing the relaxation response of the nervous system. Researchers also note that people with higher HRV (which reflects safe vagal tones) showed lower biomarkers of pressure, increased physical and psychological tolerance and better cognitive function. Heavy, abdominal breathing was also shown to minimize the' defense or flight' response during stressful situations. Many people inhale air 10-14 times a minute, so they have a shallow breathing. Ideally, air should be inhaled 6 times a minute.

In addition, the diaphragmic breathing stimulates the vagus nerve and interprets it as necessary to relax, even if this order has not been expressly provided by the nerve. The process is similar for which you feel short light bursts as you close your eyes and click your fingertips on your eyes because the brain interprets them as well.

Through diaphragmic breathing, we breathe deeply and bring oxygen to the lower part of the lungs, correctly use the diaphragm and promote relaxation. Another very successful method for vagal stimulation also requires deep breathing.

9. *Exercise* — Exercise increases the growth hormone of your brain, stimulates mitochondria of your brain, and helps to reverse mental decline. Nevertheless, Vagus nerve, which contributes to beneficial effects for the brain and mental health, has also been activated. Moderate exercise frequently increases bowel drainage through the Vagus nerve.

Laughter activates the nerve of the Vagus and increases HRV in the band.

10. *Coffee Enemas* - Enemas are like Vagus nerve sprints. Expanding the intestine increases the

activation of the vagus nerve, as with the enemas. The cleaning is achieved by increasing the liver's ability to detoxify and bind toxins in the blood. The liver is purified by releasing the toxic bile into the small, then large intestine for evacuation. The whole blood supply circulates every three minutes through the liver. If coffee is held for 12-15 minutes, blood flows four to five times for purification, much like dialysis. The coffee's water content induces intestinal peristalsis and helps flush the large intestine with the poisonous bile.

11.   ***Nervana*** - This wearable device transmits a gentle electrical wave across the left eye duct to activate the body's vagus nerve while synchronizing with music, which activates the release of neurotransmitters throughout the brain to produce a soothing sensation throughout the body.

12.   ***Relax*** – The first thing that helps maintain the Vagus nerve tone is to know how to relax.

According to Hoffman, the vagus nerve is activated by most calming activities.

In the end, the most important results can be found here.

13. ***Coughing or tensioning the muscles of the abdomen*** - When you bear down, you activate the vagus nerve as if you were passing the intestines. That's why after a bowel movement you can feel relaxed.

Thus, it stimulates your Vagus nerve if you use the bowel movement muscles.

14. ***Works on Gut Head*** - Vagus nerve impulses flow from the intestine to the brain. This was associated with the control of mood and certain kinds of fear and anxiety. A sign of good vagal tone is somebody who is under stress–an attribute that most entrepreneurs can use!

The vagus nerve constantly sends information to the brain via different nerves about the state of the body's organs, digestive tract, heart rate and other information. Studies has shown that our intestinal bacteria and brain pathways are intertwined. The gut microbiota is also believed to be the possible primary modulator of the immune and nervous systems. Keeping your gut healthy is therefore the Vagus " hack.'

Gut health varies from person to person and depends on how you are created, but generally you can: take probiotics, eat a healthy, balanced diet of full food, avoid unnecessary use of antibiotics, and moderate use of sugar or alcohol. In addition, while probiotics are still being studied for their effectiveness, an active PTSD treatment has been identified in a Canadian study. There are also implications of stress management–it can be a simple step to consider whether you can benefit from stress.

CHAPTER 4:
VAGUS NERVE FOR REDUCING INFLAMMATION

Linkage Between Stress, Inflammation And The Immune System

The vagus nerve (Crane Nerve X) is the main nerve of the autonomous nervous system's parasympathetic division (rest and digestion). It is an essential way of communication between the heart, cardiovascular system, digestive system and immune system. This bi-directional nervous path passes through the chest and abdomen and is connected to several organs.

The body is closely linked and the Vagus nerve plays a major role in organizing interaction. Signals from the brain are conveyed to the chest and abdominal organ and back to the central nervous system from the intestines and lungs. The Vagus nerve helps to create this communication network by signalling the brain to produce neurotransmitters and hormones, to organize reactions, to regulate stress reactions and to keep inflammation under control.

In controlling the parasympathetic rest, for instance, the vagus nerve plays a central role in helping to regulate breathing and heart rate, promote relaxation, stimulate digestion and create a sense of peace and calmness. The Vagus nerve releases neurotransmitters acetylcholine to help coordinate this calming reaction, which tends to be a significant brake on inflammation in the corpse.

VAGAL TONE AND ITS BENEFITS

Since it is a major control center for the body, this nerve's health is of utmost importance to your brain, your immune system and your overall inflammatory condition.

Many individuals have more vagus nerve function than others, allowing their bodies to relax after stress more quickly. Your Vagus response's intensity is known as vagal tone.

Low vagal tone with chronic inflammation was associated. Research shows that the cardiac amplitude, an indicator of reduced vagal tone, is often decreased in inflammatory conditions such as arthritis and other autoimmune diseases. This decreased vagal tone allows proinflammable cytokines (inflammatory substances that damage other cells and tissues) to become more active, leading to systemic inflammation, which leads to greater sympathetic nervous system activity and stress hormones.

Abdominal Massage As A Natural Anti-Inflammatory

Luckily, this nerve can be activated and your vagal tone improved by natural therapies, which help balance your immune system, relaxed body and mind, and lower inflammation. Research demonstrates that the Vagus nerve stimulation acts as a natural anti-inflammatory and calming agent, as it decreases the development of pro-inflammatory cytokines and calms the nervous system.

A method of self-abdominal massage is an evolving technique for reducing inflammation and tone of the vagus nerve. Gentle pressure massage has been shown to stimulate the vagus nervous system, increase digestive movements and content, and boost insulin secretion in pre-term infants to regulate their blood sugar (adult trials are still required). The combination of manual handling and stimulation of the Vagus nerve can have strong anti-inflammatory advantages.

How to Carry out Abdominal Massage

This abdominal massage technique is simple to do at home in just a few minutes. This procedure is best performed on an empty stomach a few hours after eating. Start slowly and see the reactions of your body.

1.   Lie on a soft floor mat or on a mattress.

2.   Place your hand under your breastbone or sternum. Make gentle motions downward — drive your hand down to the abdomen. Do this step a few minutes, cycle one hand over the other in a reverse motion like bicycle pedaling.

3.   First, make small circular motions on your abdomen with your fingertips. Begin to massage the sides of your abdomen and slowly move

back and forth. Go deeper and deeper with a strong yet relaxed pressure. For a few minutes, start this abdominal massage.

4. Finish your practice with a gentle, reclining two-knee spinal twist (*Supta Matsyendrasana*) for some minutes. The restorative yoga pose increases the digestion and encourages an opening of the fascia and diaphragm to help you deepen your breath.

    - Lying on your back, exhale softly into a floor or mattress as you press your lower back.

    - Breathe a few moments here as you open your lower back.

    - When ready, gently relax the abdominal muscles and bend your knees to the chest.

    - Breathe out , then lower your arms to the floor, even with your back, with your hands at your side.

- As you inhale slowly, raise your feet a little higher than your knees and slowly exhale both legs toward the floor toward the left.

- Keep your knees and your feet and knees lined together at the bottom of your hips. Remain 30 to 60 seconds in this position.

- Begin to breathe deeply and steadily, as you softly move with your breath from side to side.

Try this simple practice for your Vagus nerve power. Carryout the following exercises once or twice a day for several weeks for a few minutes. The benefits of lower pressure, enhanced digestion, better detoxification, reduced pain and squelched inflammation can surprise you!

VAGUS NERVE STIMULATION (VNS) FOR DEPRESSION AND FLOW STATE

Vagus nerve stimulation has been proven to help most people to overcome feelings of anxiety and flow state. I am so passionate about this field of work because it can be the key to opening the door to a newly found liberation for those who struggle on a physical, mental and emotional basis.

It's all about how we think at an emotional level, how we interact with others and how successful we can be. It also has a crucial impact on our physical health.

The vagus nerve stretches from the brain stem to the lower abdomen's viscera and touches almost all organs. This is related to the autonomous nervous system: an unconscious mechanism that is unintended.

The "ZONE" you are in affects a great deal on the filter you use to experience the world. Whether you feel anxious or comfortable, if your body is tense or relaxed, if your mind is thinking or calm, and if you are able to think clearly, how things taste, smell and sound.

Neuroception refers to the way we test for danger. Our nervous system talks if you encounter someone, something like; are you safe or are you dangerous? If we have a deadline, our nervous system will check for our danger to our safety.

Neuroception is automatic and rapid and will be affected by the fitness and variation of our Vagus Nerve. In how we see the world and have three regions, our autonomic state is the most important thing.

Green zone is our safe zone, where every other social engagements can take place.

- Heart rate slows down
- Stimulation of saliva and digestion
- Activation of facial muscles for connection
- Improved vocal and eye contact for connection
- Muscles in the center of the ear turn on to raise the mid-range volume to hear others ' voices.
- Essentially in this zone, our sense of sight, smell, sound, and vision change so that we are prepared for digestion and engagement.

The Yellow Zone is the state of danger: Fight-and-Flight: do I run or fight, like hell?

- Heart rate increases
- Flat and smooth facial effect
- Auditory system changes: muscles in the center of the ear shift to help distinguish low frequency noises and high frequency sounds for attackers.
- Pupils dilate
- Blood moves away from the digestive system.

The Red Zone is the Life-threatening zone (The Freeze Zone)

This is the peak where the nervous system feels they will die and immobilization takes place. It's known as death pretenders and it is the reptilian response that needs to be seen with this eye, the oldest part of our brain and injury. It is not to run but to freeze the one common response to traumatic events. We are disassociated or shut down and this is entirely unintentional.

Healthy people can easily switch between the green and the yellow system, which is why the vagus nerve is so significant. It is a challenge to know whether there is security or danger and to send that message to every organ in the body so that they are able to answer in kind.

80 percent of your Vagus nerve fibers descend to your organs and say safety or danger and 20 percent reassert safety or danger to reinstate the data.

The Vagus Nerve functions as a neural brake-so that the body slows down when it acts in the green zone.

The Vagus nerve has a second branch that functions as a buffer, but is connected to life-threatening incidents. In comparison to the green region that slows you to relax, it slows you to dissociate, causing people to freeze or dissociate themselves and what is turned on in traumatic situations. It's like the freezes reptile.

After a traumatic event, many people ask: why did I freeze? Because your nervous system chose to die and you had no control.

Why does it all look, smell and taste different? Because it is linked to any device in your body based on what you've done.

Why am I still worried? Anxiety is an overactive mechanism of neuroception where the body interprets threats where no threat is present. And we're wired like that. We have a NERVOUS system-we are negatively influenced by risk and need it to survive. We are searching for danger.

In the olden days, we referred to danger by lions chasing us. Today, it means missing a deadline or some sorts of appointments, but these same neural pathways are activated and you feel frightened.

Even in non-frightening cases, our body responds to the same neutral pathways, such as missing a train or that are late for an appointment or traffic, our body is on the same neural pathways that once have been reserved for "I don't have enough food to survive," and you always feel like crap.

The body tends to overestimate the risk of this' nerve' process.

Why does trauma last so long and why is it so hard to treat? Trauma is physiological, not psychological. Trauma is a sort of rearrangement of how the whole body works. It is not enough just to view it as a question of feeling bad and getting something to conquer. And this is the case for a lot of issues, such as anxiety, borderline personality disorder.

Low Vagal Tone

Feeling safe and in the green zone is crucial.

- This takes us to the flow state to enhance critical thinking, productivity, and learning.
- This activates healthy and beneficial hormones
- Makes life easier and more enjoyable.
- Allows the movement of the body. Most people with trauma are suffering from IBS. This doesn't make no sense from a logical point of view, but from the nervous system we see that all these are connected by the vagus nerve together. Good health is fully associated with the vagus nerve.
- This makes people like you because, thanks to mirror neurons, we are prepared for connection in the green zone.
- It optimizes the entire human experience.

The condition in which we find ourselves mostly will impact our entire human experience: the way we feel within ourselves, our emotional responses, our ability to connect with the ones we love, our ability to work and develop.

Healthy people can easily switch between the green and yellow system and that is why the vagus nerve is so critical and why I think stimulation of the vagus nerve is necessary during long periods of stress. It's a challenge to tell whether protection or danger exists and give this message to every organ in the body in order to answer in the same way.

VAGUS NERVE STIMULATION (VNS) FOR DEPRESSION

This is surgical process that can be used in treating people with treatment-resistant depression. The implanted device like a pacemaker is connected to a relaxing wire which is threaded along the nerve called the vagus nerve. The vagus nerve passes up the neck to the brain, linking regions that are supposed to be part of the mood regulation. When implanted, this system provides the vagus nerve with daily electrical impulse.

How Vagus Nerve Stimulation Works

Once the VNS operation is completed, a little battery-powered device will be inserted into your neck-the size of a silver dollar. It acts as a pacemaker. Another incision is made at the left side of the neck, and a thin wire (located just below the skin) runs from the apparatus to the major vagus nerve. The machine sends electric pulses into the nerve, transmitting them into the brain.

Such electrical pulses transmitted via the vagus nerve to the brain may alleviate the symptoms of depression for reasons that doctors do not fully comprehend. Impulse can influence how nerve cell circuits transmit signals in mood-affecting parts of the brain. However, it takes a few months before you feel the effects, though.

If applicable, the system settings (essentially dose change) in the office with a programming wall can be changed by the doctor. The system is usually set to go off periodically. You can also disable it with a special magnet.

Research on the effect of VNS on people with clinical depression has been generally positive. A research in 2005 compared 124 people who were receiving usual treatment with 205 people who received usual treatment plus VNS. Biological psychiatryin The hybrid treatment group showed more progress than the normal treatment group after one year of treatment. Among 27% of patients who received VNS, there was a significant improvement compared to 13% who did not. VNS is not fast anxiety treatment. Studies show that a treatment response can take up to 9 months on average.

VNS Risks and Side Effects

This include, cough, brief hoarseness, or shortness of breath may have side effects of the VNS. Most of these side effects arise in the 30 seconds on which the stimulator is triggered. The implantation process, like any operation, poses some risks of infection. Unlike pacemakers, when it is used out, you will finally require surgery to replace the plug. Additionally, while uncommon, system or lead damage may require additional surgery before the battery is replaced.

As the VNS system may interfere with mammograms, special positioning may be necessary to obtain the best possible image. Other medical procedures, such as heart defibrillation and ultrasound, may also affect the VNS system. Therefore, special precautions may be required before an MRI scan, so make sure your doctor knows.

You will probably continue other therapies for your anxiety, such as depression and counseling, even when you are treated with VNS.

VAGUS NERVE STIMULATION THERAPY FOR PTSD

Researchers at the University of Dallas, Texas are studying how moderate vagus nerve stimulation can help alleviate the symptoms of post-traumatic stress disorder (PTSD).

The vagus nerve regulates the sympathetic nervous system which tracks a vast range of essential bodily functions, including digestion and heart rate slowing. Vagus nerve stimulation (VNS) has been shown to enhance memory retention as a treatment for conditions including epilepsy and depression.

The effect of the technique on memory is essential: UT Dallas researchers theorized that it could help people with PTSD effectively resolve the fear response in circumstances that are not threatened.

UT Dallas scientists found that moderate electrical pulses to the vagus nerve also had some effects on defense against PTSD symptoms in a recent preclinical study published in the journal Translational Psychiatry.

"We found evidence that a treatment for traumatic memory has brought significant changes to other symptoms of PTSD, such as anxiety, agitation and avoidance," Dr Christa McIntyre, Associate Professor of Neuroscience at the Brain and Behavioral University, and the senior author of the study, said.

In mice with PTSD symptoms, scientists applied painless electric stimulation to the vagus nerve. Such signs included responses to fear and anxiety in conditions without risks and reduced social experiences.

After VNS, there were reduced responses to fear and social interaction in animals, indicating that therapy was effective in reducing symptoms of PTSD. When VNS is the same advantage to humans, the latest treatments can be effective supplementary, said Dr. Michael Kilgard, neuroscience professor at UT Dallas, and study writer.

"Such therapies commonly in use for PTSD patients include speech therapy and exposure therapy, which can help, but understandably patients do not always pursue such interventions as they do not want to undergo more trauma," said Margaret Fonde Jonsson Professor, Kilgard. "We wanted to explore ways to improve sensitivity and effectiveness of the therapy." Kilgard explained that changes for people with PTSD may not be long-lasting though they are faithful to current treatments. If you encounter a new tragedy in your life, for instance, death in the family, you usually lose a lot of your gains instead of having mild declines in PTSD symptoms.

"In our study, we found that VNS not only strengthened the reaction of fear in non-stressful situations, but also persisted after another traumatic experience," said Kilgard.

Researchers also found that VNS therapy provided protection after full discontinuation of treatment.

"We were excited to discover that there were protective effects after one week of no VNS therapy at all," said Lindsey Noble, lead author and doctoral student at UT Dallas. "We really want to know more about this and see if VNS can provide more benefits for other conditions, such as obsessive compulsive disorders and dependence across the board."

VAGUS NERVE STIMULATION THERAPY FOR ADDICTION

VNS therapy may help addicts in overcoming substance abuse, according to an effective preclinical review, which is the extinction of conditioned drug-seeking behaviors.

In the January issue of Learning and Memory, the new report "Vagus Nerve Stimulation Reduces cocaine quest and age plastics in the network extinction" has been released.

While this is an experimental study, researchers believe that their results can potentially be applied to people battling drug addiction and substance-abuse disorders. VNS treatment for certain disorders, including clinical depression, epilepsy and inflammation, has already been approved by the FDA.

The new research contributes to an increasing number of data on the advantages of VNS therapy. For example, February 2016 study found that VNS therapy enhanced default mode network connectivity which decreased Major Depressive Disorders (MDD) symptoms.

Furthermore, a research by neuroscientists and immunologists conducted in July 2016 found that VNS therapy blocked the "inflammatory reflex" by blocking pro-inflammatory cytokines output. This research was the first human study to reduce rheumatoid arthritis symptoms by causing a chain reaction that reduces cytokine levels and inflammation.

Researchers at Dallas School of Behavioral and Brain Sciences at the University of Texas found, during the new January 2017 report, that lab rats who became cocaine users decreased their drug-seeking behavior dramatically when treated with VNS therapy.

Researchers found that VNS therapy has induced improvements in synaptic plasticity in cocaine-addicted laboratory rats between prefrontal cortex and amygdala. VNS seemed to promote the "extinction training" of drug-seeking habits by increasing cravings and encrypting new reward behaviors in place of former drug-induced lever-related ones to get a cocaine hit.

In Latin, vagus means "wandering". The vagus nerve is also referred to as the "wandering nerve," because it has many branches which are different from the cerebellum's thick stems (Latin for "small brain") and the brainstem that wanders to the lowest viscera of the abdomen, which are affecting your heart and most of your major organ. The vagus nerves are a central player in the "good brain axis." In 1921, a nobel laureate German physiologist, Otto Loewi, noticed that vagus stimulation decreased the heart rate by inducing the release of the substance he called Vagusstoff. The "vagus material," later identified by scientists as acetylcholine, was the first neurotransmitter ever to be detected.

Vagus substance (acetylcholine) is like a tranquilizer which can be offered easily by taking quick, slow diaphragm breaths. Tapping your vagus nerve's energy actively could lead to inner relaxation while reducing stress and taming your inflammatory reflex at a neurobiologic stage.

The vagus nerve is the primary component of the parasympathetic nervous system which controls the response of "rest and digest" and "tend and mate." On the reverse side, the sympathetic nervous system encourages "fight or flight" response to preserve homeostasis.

A slight increase in heart rate as you inhale and a drop in the heart rate as you exhale are the natural indications for a healthy vagal tone. A higher vagal tone index is associated with positive emotions and psychological balance, which triggers an upward spiral of well-being. In addition, a low vagal tone index is associated with floating anxiety, stress, inflammation, and depression that can lead to a declining spiral of well-being.

Vagus Nerve Stimulation Can Decrease Drug Addictions via Synaptic Plasticity

The latest research on VNS therapy shows the potential to decrease drug addictions by enhancing the functional connection between Prefrontal Cortex (PFC) and Basi-Lateral Amygdala (BLA) by stimulating the vagus nerve with a mild electric current. Immunohistochemistry has been used by researchers to track changes in the PFC and BLA, which function to control cue learning and extinction.

Drug and alcohol abuse disorders typically cause PFC and other brain regions changes that affect the inhibitory regulation of drug-seeker behavior. To eradicate hardwired addictive behavior patterns, researchers at UT Dallas found that it is necessary to break the paired relationship between drug-associated indices and pay for extinction which fuels dependence during a learning phase.

Senior author of this research Sven Kroener summarized his team's results in a declaration at the University of Texas in Dallas today: "We are researching extinction training and how vagus nerve stimulation may help subjects develop a New Behavior which opposes a current, maladaptive behavior like narcotics. However, the extinction of drug-seeking memories and extinction of fearful memories rely on the same pathway/substrate in the brain. In our research, vagus nerve stimulation take into consideration the two extinction learning process and reduces the relapse as well."

This technique can really become a treatment during recovery, where people are doing these exposure treatments, looking at the triggers that caused their desire when abstaining from a safe situation. The VNS therapy can reinforce this abstinence and wean them away from drug-related activity and protect them from cravings.

You also research how distinctly activated nerves can help treat post-traumatic stress disorder (PTSD), depression, tinnitus, and help people recover from stroke paralysis. Perhaps their latest findings on the possible use of VNS therapy in human clinical trials will soon be.

CHAPTER 5:
VAGUS NERVE STIMULATION AND SOME OF ITS BENEFITS

Current VNS care patient use Epilepsy affects 1% of the U.S. population and costs $12 billion dollars (2008 figures). VNS was first used by JL Corning in the early 1880s to treat epilepsy, who felt that seizures were caused by a switch in cerebral blood flow. The first permanent implantable stimulator was used to treat drug-resistant epilepsy in 1988.In 1997, the stimulator was approved by the FDA to treat partial onset seizures which were pharmacologically resistant. The current implantable treatment system Livanova © (formerly Cyberonics) consists of a small battery-powered stimulator requiring battery removal and replacement every 6 years. The electrode with fine wire spreads from the device and is usually wrapped around the left cervical Vagus.

Case reports indicate that the right Vagus may be used in conditions in which it is not advised to use the left

Vagus. Since the right Vagus internalizes the sinoatrial node, the ECG monitoring is best used to activate the right. The system can be disabled for 30–90 seconds to give the Vagus a short stimulus. Once the system is implanted, it is programmed by a physician using a microcomputer, but when they experience a seizure, patients may alter the stimulus program as appropriate. In hospitals worldwide, over 100,000 VNS implants were implanted (as of 2015). Dysphony, hoarseness, and cough are the most common side effects recorded. All can be mitigated by adjusting stimulus parameters. Nevertheless, standard treatment for epilepsy and depression requires a stimulation range of 20–30 HZ, a pulsing period of up to 500 microseconds and a stimulation time of 30–90 seconds accompanied by off-time stimulation of 5 minutes.

Data collected during the first decade of clinical VNS was successful in patients with pharmacored seizures. Following 2–3 years of treatment, nearly 40% of the patients with VNS had a 50% decrease in seizures. The mechanisms through which VNS contributes to changes in neurochemistry and prevents epileptic seizures are still not understood, although there is some evidence that Vagus nerve is effective in quenching seizures in regions that can be more exciting. Both areas are limbic, thalamic and thalamocortic projections. VNS can also affect midbrain and back-brain structures that can lead to the suppression of seizures, although the specific changes on these cortical circuits remain unknown.

VNS also enhances the activation of locus and raphe nuclei, and reduces downstream norepinephrine and serotonin releases, both of which have proven antiepileptic effects. The effectiveness of VNS in treating refractive epilepsy with few side effects supports its extension to additional conditions as well as to larger populations. VNS may also be useful to treat mothers with medical epilepsy. For one study, the risk of death during pregnancy for women with epilepsy was significantly higher compared with women without epilepsy. The goal is to improve seizure control and reduce utero fetal exposure to anti-epileptic drugs which are correlated with significant congenital malformations, delayed growth and neurocognitive deficits during the perinatal era.

VNS was successfully used in women who had pregnant women as a treatment for medally refractive epilepsy, and physicians concluded that VNS is a viable option for pregnancy treatment. VNS appears to be effective as a non-pharmacological therapy in the expecting mother for seizure control, and no clear evidence of harm to the fetus which grows. No major clinical trials to determine whether the VNS has a long-term impact on the developing fetus have been conducted to date.

Epilepsy affects 0.5%–1% or about 470,000 children in the pediatric population. Severe epileptic seizures can have a profound impact on the long-term neuroscience and social outcome of children and on their families. Effective treatment may improve the quality of life of adolescents, because children with epilepsy often have psychological and cognitive problems and as adults have bad social effects. Antiepileptic drugs have high side effects and can adversely affect children's behavior. This implies that there is a high risk of psychological and psychiatric disturbance even in children with more easily controlled epilepsy. Beninous rolandic epilepsy and absence of epilepathy have been more violent, stressful and anxious than epilepsy-free kids.

Continuing research concentrate on noninvasive approaches in pediatric patients for epilepsy diagnosis. This includes a study conducted by the Chinese Academy of Medical Sciences to test a less invasive, non-implant transcutaneous auricular Vagus nerve stimulator as effective pediatric epilepsy treatment.

The research investigates improvements in seizure frequency and variability in the heart rate, quality of life and electroencephalogram at 2, 4 and 6 months after stimulation. The effects of VNS on 141 boys, 61% < 12 years of age, was examined in a retrospective cohort study by Elliott et al. Researchers concluded that VNS in children under 12 years old was as successful and relatively free from complications as it was in older pediatric patients. In this study the incidence of seizures in these children also declined significantly, from an average of 10 to 3 a week. In 41% of patients, the rate of seizures decreased by 75%. Symptoms of VNS occurred in a small percentage of children with hoarseness (0.7%), cough (0.7%) and low arm pain (0.5%). Hallböök et al found that pediatric VNS responses were similar to adult responses. However, In 40% of children implanted with VNS stimulators, the seizure rate was decreased by 50 percent. Retrospective findings of 75 children with epileptic disorder found that only 5.4 percent of patients experienced adverse effects such as hoarseness, cough, and drooling, in which all are reversible with stimulation parameter changes.

Neonates may also benefit from a non-pharmacological approach to epilepsy control. Phenobarbital and levetiracetam are currently available for prescription epilepsy treatment in neonates, although each may have harmful side effects. Phenobarbital is the most widely used neonatal anti-epileptic but can have both behavioral and respiratory side effects. The psychological side effects of levetiracetam. While VNS is approved for FDA only in children over 12 years of age, along with anti-epileptic medication, it is used for children under 1 year of age. A research by Fernandez et al. in children < 3 years of age indicated that VNS is effective in children with medically insensitive epilepsy. In their study, VNS resulted in a 33% reduction in patients ' seizure rate and the disease epilepticus was no longer a symptom after 1 year of treatment. Moreover, regular MRIs are associated with a lower incidence of seizure.

Medically refractive epilepsy is more likely to occur in children with developmental disabilities or autism. One study estimated that 5 to 38 percent of children with autism suffer from epilepsy. A research by Kirchberger et al indicated that VNS induced a decrease of 50% in the rate of seizures in 61% of developmentally delayed patients. Levy et al. also discovered that there was no statistically significant difference in the advantages of seizure reduction and improvements in quality of life between refractory patients with autism or autism. Based on these results, VNS tends to be a safe and effective therapy for pediatric patients with epilepsy.

Depression Treatment

Severe or chronic depression affects up to 1.5% of the general population and many of these patients get little medical relief. In 2000, unemployment in the United States was estimated at $83.1 billion. Of these, $26.1 billion was spent on direct education, $51.5 billion was spent on indirect labor, and $5.4 billion was spent on suicide related mortality. Although the VNS was not originally developed for treating depression, mood changes were observed in patients with VNS in order to treat epilepsy. The FDA approved recurrent or persistent depression medication for VNS in 2005. VNS therapy has been licensed for patients aged 18 years who had at least one major depressive episode and failed to respond correctly to one of four separate prescription antidepressant therapies. A major depressive episode is defined as having five out of nine depressed symptoms, including depression in the mood and lack of concern for normal daily life, occurring almost daily for at least 2 weeks, as the Diagnostic and Statistical Manual for Mental Disorders (DSM-IV). The goal of this procedure is to restore everyday function and prevent recurrence and recovery as well as relieve current symptoms, in which VNS has been shown to be successful in a broad spectrum of patients. In a study conducted by Bajbouj, VNS was received in patients with chronic "refractory therapy," in which 53.1% of patients met the Hamilton Rating Scale on Depression (HRSD28) (the most used symptom gravity scale) response criterion. Moreover, 38.9 percent met the remittance criteria with HRSD scores < 10.

Depression is often difficult to treat and patients with repeated depressive periods treated with traditional medications often have recurrence or not truly recovery. Depression is often difficult to treat. A research by Nahas et al revealed chronic or persistent major depressive VNS-receiving conditions that may have beneficial long-term effects. 42 percent of their patients had a positive effect in their study and 22 percent saw their recovery two years later. Both Bajbouj et al and Nahas et al use the same definition for clinically significant remission that are characterized as the absence of serious symptoms of depression. Results of neuroimaging studies show that VNS stimulation improves the mood-enhancing advantages of medial and prefrontal cortical transmission. These regions include neurons that release both anticonvulsant and antidepressant neurotransmitters, such as serotonin and norepinephrine Although VNS is unlikely to be used as a' first-order' or primary depression medication, current clinical evidence suggests progress in its use as alternative treatment for chronic refractory depression.

Around 6 and 13 percent of pregnant women experience depression symptoms during and after delivery. The most commonly prescribed medications for women with depression are selective serotonin reuptake inhibitors (SSRIs), although the safety of SSRI therapy in the fetus remains unanswered. Antidepressants may lead to low birth weight and premature delivery during pregnancy as they may pass through the placenta. A Husain et al case report showed that VNS is an effective treatment for depression and delivery during pregnancy, with no adverse effects on a mother or fetus. A recent work on a VNS rat model shows no significant VNS effect on pups born to a dam with an implanted VNS stimulator. Preliminary research indicates that VNS can be beneficial to both mother and fetus, although more research is necessary to provide a clearer picture of the effects.

While depression also affects many teens, there are limited treatment options for pediatric patients. Longitudinal studies on children with major depressive disorders showed that the repetition rate is 40% within two years and 70% within five years. Most children undergoing major depression are diagnosed with psychotherapy, but in contrast to treatment, their depressive symptoms continue. As with pregnant mothers, the most common antidepressant drugs used in pediatrics are SSRI.48 Studies in pediatric patients with VNS implants for the treatment of epilepsy have shown improvement in mood, as have adults diagnosed with VNS. A Hallbök and al research found that seizures were not only reduced in children with epilepsy treated with VNS but also that adherence and mood were increased while depressive symptoms were decreased. Twelve of the 15 children studied had their quality of life improved. More studies are required to investigate the effect of VNS on pediatric depression, but the preliminary data indicate that it remains promising and can give children with depression long-term benefits.

Potential uses and mechanisms of VNS

As a counter-inflammatory treatment, an exciting new application is VNS. Inflammation is involved in a number of chronic diseases, including heart, arthritis and Alzheimer's. Preliminary preclinical evidence shows that the VNS can relieve inflammatory responses by triggering the CAP–a long line from Vagus afferents through the autonomous brain stem and forebrain cortical structures, and then back through the descending Vagus efferents. The CAP upregulates HMGB1, which can control the expression of cytokine leading to anti-inflammatory effects. In recent years, Tracey et al. have made considerable efforts to quantify VNS's function as an anti-inflammatory regulator, mainly by modifying acetylcholine control. Such results show clearly that Vagus nerve stimulation plays a major role in peripheral cholinergic release and its supposed role in the regulation of inflammation. The CAP also affects nicotinic acetylcholine receptor acetylcholine levels (nAChRs). A number of new and ongoing research concentrate on the impact of VNS on inflammatory conditions such as RA, Crohn's disease, bowel syndrome and fibromyalgia. Additional studies concentrate on how VNS causes brain trauma and stroke. As these are continuous trials, the effectiveness of VNS therapy is currently unknown for these conditions. Lots of the inflammatory disorders that VNS may treat affect the pediatric and newborn population as well. Since VNS has proved effective in epilepsy and anxiety for adults and pediatric populations, it is appropriate for VNS therapy to be beneficial for younger patients with a range of conditions, although limited data are available on pediatric applications. Nonetheless, these summary results provide strong justification for extending the research into the applications of VNS as anti-inflammatory treatment for a variety of different inflammatory diseases.

Sepsis

Sepsis is typically due to systemic bacterial infections and persistent activation of the pro-inflammatory cytokine cascades, a multibillion dollar health burden. Sepsis costs $22,000 per patient and affects up to 18 million people every year. Kessler et al used vagotomized mouse to demonstrate that a lack of Vagus CNS inputs can bring about an adverse outcomes in a murine model of stent peritonitis in colon ascends. Tumor necrosis factor α (TNFα) in an ex vivo culture of kupffer cells was decreased in the vagotomised mouse in contrast with controls, even when stimulated with lipopolysaccharide (LPS). Huang et al. have shown that VNS has helped to attenuate inflammation by restoring the balance between sympathetic and parasympathetic tones and thus preventing sepsis. These researchers used an inflammation intravenous LPS injection method for induce sepsis. However, the cardiovascular variety was decreased in addition to the decrease in ACh in the LPS + VNS treatment group down to baseline levels, compared with elevated levels in the LPS-only community. Borovikova et al. used VNS in a similar model of LPS-induced endotoxemia and observed reduced mortality due to vagally mediated release of acetylcholine.

Limiting inflammation in patients with no drugs is important because the neonates, particularly preterm infants, are more susceptible to sepsis because of their underdeveloped immune systems and susceptibility to perinatal infection (chorioamnionitis, etc). Since VNS appears to regulate inflammations by modulating the cytokine cascade, our laboratory is investigating the impact of VNS in respiratory control regions of the brain stem, interleukin-6(IL-6), TNFα and IL-1β, on early pro-inflammatory cytokines. We looked at the NTS and the hypoglossal motor nucleus (XII), regions of critical importance for breathing regulation, which are a model for preterm infants for breathing problems in neonatal rats. In this study, we show that VNS reducesIL-6 and TNFα expression in response to a short

(30-minute) high-frequency VNS stimuli. We hope that this preclinical translation can lead eventually to minimally invasive VNS therapy so that early intervention and the risk of septic sepsis can be minimized among preterm infants.

The amount of time that VNS takes to be successful and the invasive aspect of implantation are two important concerns in applying VNS to neonatal care. While it may take months to show dramatic effects to have currently used VNS for epilepsy and depression, a short-term stimulation has been used to quickly reduce inflammation, and our research has shown that a single end of high-frequency stimulation (30 minutes) could work as an anti-inflammation treatment. Transcutaneous stimulation was also used to treat depression and headaches which show efficacy even in short-term applications with surface electrodes. A He et al study uses transcutaneous cervical or auricular Vagus stimulation to treat epilepsy effectively. Lots studies will be needed to determine whether the combination of high frequency stimulation and transcutaneous stimulation is an effective treatment for neonatal inflammatory disorders. Preliminary work by Wilson

Laboratory and others suggests that VNS treatment in neonates can and will be useful.

Pain management

VNS systems are also common for chronic or intermittent pain disorders such as fibromyalgia and migraines. Pain management Lange et al. conducted a phase I / II clinical study to assess VNS as an additional treatment for fibromyalgia patients due to their effects on serotonergic and noradrenergic neural circuits–all involving experiences of pain. Our hypothesis is based on the results of patients who reported reduced pain perception with depression treated with VNS. Lange et al's study included 12 females with fibromyalgia with the same stimulation parameters as epilepsy care. After 10 months, 7 of the patients had the small medical difference (MCID+) that they considered effective in their VNS pain symptoms.

One chronic pain condition promising for VNS diagnosis is migraine headaches. In a report by Barbanti et al, 50 patients with migraine obtained externally administered VNS therapies in two 120-second intervals of 3 minutes between them. Of these patients,

56 percent reported 1 hour among pain relief, and 64 percent reported 2 hours of pain relief. The ACT1 (NCT01792817) review, a clinical trial to treat cluster headaches, was performed by Silberstein et al. Our findings indicate that episodic cluster headaches can be successfully treated with non-invasive VNS. These findings need more study and more randomized multicenter trials, but they provide promising proof that Vagus Nerve Stimulation can be used to control fibromyalgia and migraines.

Obesity

While VNS may not be prescribed as a first-line defense against obesity, research has been conducted on the impact of VNS on diet and weight to test VNS for use as a supplemental treatment for obesity regulation. It is particularly important to find alternative treatments for obesity given that 69% of adults and 20% of teenagers in the United States are overweight or obese. Burneo et al found that 62% of patients implanted with VNS had significant weight loss to control epilepsy. Bodenlos et al. conducted a study on the association between VNS and dietary cravings in depressed adults, which found that a reduced food cravings result from left cervical VNS. Recent work by Val-Laillet etcetera has shown that a persistent bilateral stimulation of the Vagus nerve triggered a lower intake of food and sweet cravings in obese minipigs. This research did not suggest that VNS induced weight loss; rather, VNS avoided excess weight gain. The results of these studies are remarkable, but it is still unclear how VNS affects weight loss. Several theories include metabolic increases, fatty processing declines, or changes in signal satiety. An alternative potential mechanical mechanism suggested for the effect of VNS on weight is decreased intestinal caloric absorption, which can be inferred on the basis that vagal tones can modify peptides to change intestinal motility and absorption. This preliminary results facilitate further work on VNS and the effects of autonomous regulation and hypothalamic signaling modulation and their interactions with the enteric nervous system.

The effect of the VNS on morbid obesity was shown in a study by Ikramuddin et al. As a major risk for bariatric surgery, researchers are looking for alternative, less invasive methods of obesity control. In contrast with placebo patients, their test showed that weight loss was more important by statistically significant margins in patients with VNS.64 More work was needed but the implantation of VNS equipment could be an attractive choice for managed weight and obesity in patients who have not progressed with conventional weight-control methods.

Cardiovascular Disease

VNS will alter cardiac control due to convergence of inputs at the autonomous brain stem control centers, but how long and to what degree is uncertain. The downward heart branch of the Vagus is essential to normal heart function. Atherosclerosis is believed to be caused by low-grade systemic inflammation, which often predisposes one to coronary heart disease. Since there are growing signs that VNS is anti-inflammatory, it can provide another way to treat heart disease and atherosclerosis. In the CARDIA 2007 survey, Sloan et al showed there is a reverse relationship, measured by heart rate variability, among inflammatory marker and vagus nervous activity which indicates that VNS is the key to anti-inflammatory sound. Researchers also suggest that high levels of pro-inflammatory markerslikeIL-6 and the C-reactive protein can indicate a coronary artery disease predisposition. VNS can also provide a therapeutic treatment for heart failure prevention. Zhang et al. used a canine model to show that chronic VNS leads to the regulation of cardiac rate and increases heart function in a high-quality ventricular system. Zhao et al showed in a model of rat ischemia / reperfusion (I / R) that the VNS enhanced heart function and decreased the infarction volume. It also showed that VNS reduced mesenteric artery pathology and vasodilation according to the I / R template and lower TNFα and IL-1β were present in serum. It probably results in the VNS effect on release and systemic levels of acetylcholine and an upregulation of expression M3AChR / a7nAChr, which were involved in inflammatory modulation (see "Potential uses and mechanisms of the VNS section"). Chapleau et al. used a high salt, spontaneously hypertensive rat model to demonstrate that proper VNS avoided aortic reinforcement and decreased endothelial dysfunction progression. In addition, the serum levels ofIL-6 in VNS rats were significantly higher. This could suggest that VNS modulates inflammatory activity in this extreme hypertension model. Such studies create a link between cardiovascular disease, inflammation and vagal activity that can be affected by VNS.

Lung Injury

A treatment for ventilator-induced lung injury is considered VNS (VILI) due to pressure-induced damage to lung alveoli. Inflammation has shown that VILI is more likely to occur, often caused by serious lung infections. Substantial pulmonary inflammation can also be caused by other respiratory disorders such as acute lungs failure and acute respiratory distress syndrome, both of which can be exacerbated by sepsis. Dos Santos et al. studies have shown that the Vagus nerve plays a major role in pulmonary inflammation. Interruption of the CAP by vagotomy contributes to degradation of the VILI. Mechanical ventilation vagotomized animals had increased alveolar damage and hemorrhage levels compared with control animals. Later studies demonstrated that electrical and pharmacological VNS attenuated the lung injury in "two-hit" VILI system (inflammatory and pro-apoptotic responses, followed by high tidal pressure vent, which can further damage the lung).

VNS may also be effective in combining intestinal and pulmonary injuries. Reys et al. have shown that VNS prevents intestinal barrier failure and protects against lung injury in a study of lung injury caused by hemorrheatic shock. In addition, in a in vitro culture model of pulmonary endothelial cells, pharmacological inhibition of nicotinic cholinergic receptors indicates that VNS works by CAP to prevent lung damage and gut–barrier break-up. A Levy et al study also showed that VNS alleviated lung injury from hemorrhagic trauma by reducing intestinal permeability. Both studies show that Vagus ' nervous activity is essential for normal lung function, and it is very important for further research to use VNS to enhance lung injury outcomes. Further research is also needed to prevent gut-barrier interactions that lead to visceral inflammation.

Stroke and TBI

TBI and stroke are also causes of widespread neural inflammation that VNS can alleviate. The effect of VNS on TBI, tissue and serum ghrelin and serum TNFα have been evaluated in a study by Bansal et al. Their study was based upon the assumption that sepsis, multi-organ failure and other adverse effects could be avoided by preventing an inflammatory overshoot after TBI. Because ghrelin is regulated by acetylcholine levels, it is reasonable to assume that the VNS can use a ghrelin or other hypothalamic-gated mechanism to treat TBI. The serum TNFα, the early cytokine marker for trauma and ischemical injury was reduced by VNS. Cytokine expression control by VNS can give these patients a significant therapeutic value. As VNS is considered to be anti-inflammatory and affect acetylcholine levels, these improvements can provide an effective and controllable way to modulate injury due to stroke, ischemia or trauma in cytokine up regulation and neurotransmitters re-equilibrium.

Diabetes

One inflammatory disease that can benefit from VNS therapy is autoimmune diabetes. Recent work has shown the importance of the Vagus nerve in diabetes and other associated diseases pathophysiology, which in effect imply that the VNS may be helpful in treating these diseases. Cardiovascular risk is long associated with diabetes, but it is not understood which mechanism is used to synergize increased risk and diabetes to intensify disease. Pal et al discovered that relatives of type 2 diabetics had an increased risk of sympathovagal cardiovascular disease. Changes in the tone of sympathovagus that underlie the increased self-inflammation that can be the basis of this increased risk. Woie and Reed have shown a correlation between changes in tracheal edema, control, diabetic, and insulin-treated diabetic rats that indicates a significantly higher barrier breakdown in control animals but a decrease in diabetic rats.77 Changes in airway secretion are loosely mediated and an altered diabetes Vagus tone which worsen chronic inflammation sensitivity. The role of vagal tones in metabolism and obesity is a wider issue. In satiety and feeding behavior, vagal afferents and hypothalamus projections play an important role, and distortion of vagal afferent traffic may help prevent inflammation from obesity and down regulation of decreasing cholinergic tone. Meyers et al used selective efferent stimulation, which can be a potential treatment for type 2 diabetes, to reduce blood glucose significantly. The interaction between inflammation and metabolism is becoming clear, but further research is needed to determine the potential role of VNS in the treatment of diabetes. This Meyers et al study uses a raw method of selective active stimulation by slicing the Vagus nerve above the stimulating electrode. However, selective blocking of vagal fibers by various parameters of electrical stimulation can provide the answer to the metabolism of VNS. As Vagus nerve cutting is not an ideal solution for human patients, similar results can be obtained through the use of different parameters that can select fully stimulate fiber type or afferent / efferent traffic. Patel and Butera have obtained these results by using both Vagus and sciatic nerves in rats for high-frequency stimulation. It is still to be decided if criteria for selective stimulation, such as those used by Patel et al., can be used to replicate Meyers et al without having to isolate the Vagus nerve.

RA

RA is a autoimmune inflammatory disease of unknown origin resulting in chronic synovial inflammation and damage to bone and cartilage due to cytokine release and progressive inflammatory harm. In cells recovered from synovial fluid and synovial tissue, nicotine receptors are present alpha 7(α7), especially in cells with macrophage-like morphologies. The general suppression of cholinergic anti-inflammatory pathways is important for RA. The analysis summarizes the current literature on the role of vagus tone in RA module and the tentative evidence for further research as in so many of these inflammatory disorders. VNS devices were implanted in RA patients in a recently concluded study by SetPoint Medical Corporation. Following 6 weeks of treatment, patients were assessed and symptoms had improved by 20 percent. More studies are necessary to determine the function of VNS in RA care, in particular the possible role of VNS in cytokine cascade modulation by α7 receptors.

CHAPTER 6:
FACTORS THAT CAN STIMULATE YOUR VAGUS NERVE

Effective vagal nerve function is vital to optimum health for all, and often does not operate well in many cases of chronic disease. In this chapter, we will discuss the signs of low vagal tone, how relaxation raises the tone and how your health improves.

WAYS TO STIMULATE THE NERVE VAGUS

1. Cold

Studies have shown that your flight-or-flight mechanism decreases as your body adjusts to cold and your resting-and-digest process increases, and this is regulated by the vagus nerve.

Some form of acute cold exposure can increase the activation of the vagus nerve.

To start with, you may dip your face in cold water. I graduated from college and now take cold showers, expose myself to ice, and drink cold milk.

Cold showers and brief exposure to cold stimulate the vagus nervous system and the rest and digestion system.

2. Chanting or Singing

Singing increases the amplitude of the heart rate variability (HRV). The HRV increases slightly in different ways by humming, mantra singing, singing hymns and energetic music.

Singing starts the work of a vagal pump and sends soothing vibrations through the chorus. Also, singing at the top of lungs enables the muscles at the back of your throat to initiate the vagus.

Upbeat energetic singing stimulates your nervous system and your vagus nerve, which lets you into the flow state.

Singing in unison in churches and synagogues also enhances the function of HRV and vagus.

The singing of oxytocin was found to increase.

Choral singing, chants, and energetic singing stimulate your vagus nervousness, protect your heart and help you float.

3. Yoga

Yoga enhances the vagus nerve and general function of the parasympathic system.

A 12-week yoga procedure was associated with better mood and anxiety than a walking control group. The study found that thalamic GABA levels are increased, which are related to better mood and lower anxiety.

4. Meditation

Studies have shown that, there are two sorts of meditation can stimulate the vagus nerve. Loving-kindness meditation raises the vagus nerve tone, as measured by variability of the heart rate and Om chant.

5. Positive social relationships

In a study carried out, participants were told to sit and think passionately about others, repeating quietly phrases such as, ***"may you feel safe and happy, may you feel healthy and may you live comfortably."***

Meditators displayed an overall increase in positive emotions including happiness, curiosity, fun, serenity and hope after the class relative to the tests. This emotional and psychological shift was attributed to a stronger sense of connection to others and an increase in generally functioned through heart rate variability.

Nonetheless, actually meditating did not always lead to a more toned vagus nerve. The change occurred only in meditators who were happier and socially connected.

Those who meditated just as much but did not say that they felt close to others did not show a difference in the tone of the vagus nerve.

Meditation and social relationships strengthen the vagus nerve and cultivate happiness, serenity and empathy.

6. Slow and Deep Breathing

The vagus nerve is also stimulated by deep and slow breathing.

Heart and neck have neurons with receptors called baroreceptors which sense blood pressure and send a neuronal signal to your mind (NTS), which stimulates your vagus nerve, which allows your heart to lower blood pressure and cardiac levels. The effect is a less (sympathetic) and more rest-and-digest (parasympathetic) fight-or-flight activation.

Baroreceptors can be prone to variations. The more alert they are, the more likely they will fire and let your brain know that your blood pressure is too high and that it is time to activate the vagus nerve to will it.

Quick breathing, with a breathing time approximately equal, increases Baroreceptor tolerance and vagal activation, lowering blood pressure and reducing anxiety by reducing your compassionate nervous system and raising your parasympathic nerves.

For an average adult it can be very beneficial to breathe about 5-6 breaths per minute.

Tip: You have to breathe slowly from your stomach. Which means your belly will stretch or go out when you breathe in. You will cave in when you breathe out your stomach. The more your stomach expands and the larger it grows, the more you breathe.

Slow and deep breathing increases the function of your vagus nerves, relaxes you and lowers blood pressure. Try to get 5-6 breaths per minute from your stomach.

7. Laughter

As the popular saying "Laughter is the best medicine." Many studies have shown the health benefits of laughter. As it seems, laughter is found to stimulate the vagus nerve, and laughter therapy can be safe and beneficial to health.

A research carried out on yoga laughter showed that the laughter group has an increased HRV (heart rate variability).

There are various cases of fainting as a result of laughter, this is so because of the over-stimulation of vagus nerve / parasympathic system.

For instance, fainting can occur after laughing, urination, vomiting, chewing, and bowel movements may occur, all of which are accompanied by vague activation.

There are lots of reports of people fainting as a result of laughter with a rare disorder (Angelman's), which is associated with increased vagus stimulation.

Laughter is also sometimes a vagus nerve stimulation side effect.

A good laugh is good for cognitive function and protects you from heart disease. It also improves beta-endorphins and nitric oxide and also beneficial to the vascular system.

Laughter activates the vagus nerve and has many health benefits, including prevention of heart disease. Overdoing it, however, in rare cases can cause fainting.

8. Prayer

Studies showed that the recitation of the rosary increases the vagus stimulation. This increases cardiovascular functions like diastolic blood pressure and HRV in general.

Research also showed that reading a rosary creed takes about 10 seconds and so readers breathe in 10 seconds (includes both in and out), through the HRV and hence the vagus function.

Prayer slows and deepens the respiration which activates the nerve vagus and protects the heart.

9. PEMF

Magnetic fields can activate the vagus nerve. Studies have found that therapy with Pulsed Electromagnetic Field (PEMF) can improve heart rate variability and enhance vagus stimulation.

In my brain and my gut, I use a pulsed magnetic stimulator called ICES, which activates my vagus nerve and increases my appetite.

I recommend that you use this in your brain, gut, and side of your neck. Inflammation reduces and my gut flow increases when I fix the ICES on my gut.

At first I did not understand how it could have systemic effects if I put it on my stomach, but the main reason for this must be the vagus nerve.

PEMF therapy can improve vagus nerve function, thereby promoting heart health, inflammation reduction and digestion.

10. Breathing exercises

Strength breathing in and out would likely better activate the vagus nerve— such as backpack jogging.

A breathing exercise is to breathe as hard as possible until you feel very tired and awakening. I haven't seen research on this, yet I think it will be beneficial to your vagus nerve.

11. Probiotics

The intestinal nervous system is connected to the brain via the vagus nerve. There is an increasing evidence that that points to an effect gut microbiota has on the brain.

In a study conducted, mice augmented by probiotic **Lactobacillus rhamnosus** reported some positive changes in GABA receptors mediated by the vagus nerve in an animal study. GABA brain receptors control mood positively, a clear connection between vagus nerve intestinal stimulation by **Lactobacillus rhamnosus**. The development of evidence that probiotics may have positive health effects is accompanied by rhamnosis and enhanced GABA activities.

12. Exercise

Gentle exercise increases gut flow and this flow is regulated by the vagus nerve, which also implies that exercise activates the vagus nerve.

13. Massage

Massaging vital places such as the carotid sinus (located on your neck) can stimulate the vagus and minimize convulsions. (Note: carotid sinus massage due to possible fainting is not recommended at home). Pressure massage can stimulate your vagus nerve. Such massages help children gain weight by relaxing the intestines and are primarily activated by vagus nerve stimulation.

Foot massages may also improve your vagal movement and variability of heart rate as your heart beat rate and blood pressure decrease. All of these reduce the risk of cardiac disease. Foot, neck, and pressure massages activate the vagus nerve, help digestion and cardiac health.

14. Fasting

Reducing calories and intermittent fasting both boost the heart rate variability of the vagal tone in animals. In fact, some anecdotal reports reveal that intermittent fasting improves the variability of the heart rate. If you rapidly, part of the metabolism decrease is regulated by the vagus nerve.

The vagus senses a drop in blood glucose and electrical and chemical stimulation in the gut. It raises the vagus impulses from the liver to the brain (NTS), slowing the rate of metabolism.

Hormones such as NPY increase during fasting, while CCK and CRH decrease. If we eat, it's the reverse. Stimulatory signals of the intestine related to satiety help to improve sympathetic function and stress response (higher CRH, CCK and lower NPY).

You may be more responsive to oestrogen by the vagus nerve. Fasting increases in the number of estrogen receptors mediated by the vagus nerve in certain parts of the brain (NTS and PVN).

Fasting slows the metabolic rate by promoting slightly active nerve activity.

15. Laying or Sleeping on Your Right Side

Researches have revealed that laying or sleeping on your right side increases the variance of the heart rate and vagal stimulation more than being on other side. Laying or sleeping on your back results in the lowest vagus activation.

16. Tai Chi

Tai chi increases variability of the heart rate and thus highly likely activation of the vagus.

17. Gargling

The vagus nerve stimulates the back of your throat muscles, which makes you to gag. There is a contractions of these muscles during gargling, which activates the vagus nerve and strengthens the gastrointestinal tract. Gargle first before you swallow water.

18. Seafood (EPA and DHA)

In the lectin reduction diet, I'm a big proponent of seafood. EPA and DHA improve heart rate variability and decrease heart rate. It means that the vagus nerve is activated. As a mega-dosing test, I took ten pills of fish oil, and my heart rate dropped from 60 to 40. But fish oil really does have a lower heart rate in my self-experiments, possibly mediated in part by the vagus nerve.

19. Oxytocin

Oxytocin increases brain-to-intestinal vagal nerve activity (in the brain and orally absorbed) which induces relaxation and decreases appetite. Mice that took off their vagus did not show the oxytocin appetite-reducing effects.

20. Zinc

Zinc enhances the stimulation of vagus in rats for 3 days and supports a zinc-deficient diet. It's a very common mineral of which most people aren't getting enough.

21. Tongue Depressors

These depressors activate the gag reflex. Some people claim that, the gag reflexes are like reaching for the distinctly nerve while gagging and singing are like sprinting.

22. Acupuncture

The vagus nerve is stimulated with conventional acupuncture points, particularly around the ears.

The acupuncture is so important that a man died from too low a heart rate after vagus nerve stimulation.

23. Serotonin

The serotonin is capable of simulating vagus nerve through different receptors such as; 5HT1A, 5-HT2, 5-HT3, 5-HT4, 5-HT6. However, 5-HT7 receptors, on the other hand reduces the vagus activation. Serotonin therefore has various effects, but overall the vagus nerve should be stimulated. To raise your level of serotonin, you can take 5-HTP.

24. Chewing Gum

A gut hormone known as CCK directly stimulates vagus nerve subtly in the brain. CCK's ability to reduce food consumption and appetite relies on the vagus nerve impulse to and fro the brain. Chewing gum helps improve the production of CCK.

25. Eating Fiber

GLP-1 is a satiating hormone that activates vagus impulse to the brain, slows down intestinal/gut movements and makes you feel fuller. Fiber is a great way to increase GLP-1.

26. Enemas

The bowel expansion increases the activation of the vagus nerve, as is achieved with enemas.

27. Tensing or coughing the Stomach Muscles

At that point you are experiencing a bowel movement, you activate the vagus nerve. That's why after a bowel movement, you can feel relaxed. And, if you're using the bowel muscles, the vagus nerve will be activated.

28. Thyroid Hormones

In rats, thyroid hormones enhances their appetites and in this way the vagus nerve is stimulated.

29. Sun Exposure

In a research conducted, the Alpha-MSH prevents stroke damage in rats by activating the vagus nerve which reduces inflammation. In some cases, alpha-MSH (DMV) injection slightly excites the vagus nerve. Obviously, sun exposure improves alpha-MSH.

30. Alpha-GPC (acetylcholine)

Although I haven't seen any research enhancing Alpha-GPC itself, the main vagal neurotransmitter is acetylcholine. It means that many of the symptoms of vagal stimulation will occur.

Alpha-GPC is a great way to increase acetylcholine, but the question is not whether the vagus nerve will be stimulated.

INHIBITORS

1. Insulin (Carbohydrates)

Suppresses the vagus nerve portion of the liver and allows inflammatory molecules to come out of the liver. The function of the vagus nerve and therefore of the liver is impaired by high insulin levels seen in obesity.

2. Capsaicin

This is the most effective (and spicy) way to inhibit the nerve.

3. Ginger

Ginger helps in preventing vomiting and nausea by inhibiting the vagus nerve serotonin in the digestive tract. High-carbon foods, chili pepper and ginger can inhibit your vagus stimulation.

THE VAGUS NERVE AND HORMONES

- *Orexin*

Orexin hormones are located in centers that regulate the activation of the brain's vagus nerves.

Orexin activates the brain's vagus nerve which facilitates gut movement. The pancreas can also be stimulated. Orexin may increase the tolerance to glucose and resistance to insulin through the liver vagus nerve.

On the other hand, orexin is able to suppress the activation in competition with CCK of vagus nervous signals in the brain. Orexin can activate the brain, liver and pancreas of the vagus nerve. It increases bowel circulation and resistance to insulin.

- ***Ghrelin***

Ghrelin raises growth hormone and appetite by activating the distinctly nervous signal from the brain to the gut, and capsaicin (in chili) reduces this. Ghrelin activates the brain pancreas through the vagus.

- ***Leptin***

Vagal brain impulses are triggered by leptin. Leptin potentials CCK-inducing vagus nerve activation Leptin-resistant animals have been hungry because the vagus nerve is less prone to CCK.

Nonetheless, another study found that leptin effects do not play a major role in the intake of food.

Leptin induces satiety by activation of the vagus nerve, although this will likely not affect your intake of food.

- *CRH*

CRH has complex nerve effects. This reduces the operation from the brain to the heart. The activation of the vagus nerve slows the heart rate, but CRH reduces it and increases cardiac output.

CRH activates the brain vagus impulses to the column (through cholinergic transfer, triggering the dorsal nucleus of the vagus).

OTHER

All Stimulation of the vagus nerve normalizes an overactive nervous system.

Vagus nerve can help in reducing pain, and in certain cases, estradiol reduces pain.

In addition to influencing *oxytocin* release, the vagus nerve is essential for testosterone release. If it doesn't work well, low testosterone can be the cause.

Testosterone can make people more aggressive, but not when the vagus nerve works correctly.

A proper functioning of the vagus nerve is essential for the development of Growth Hormone-Releasing Hormone (GHRH) and IGF-1.

Certain hormones like **parathyroid hormone**, which is essential for converting vitamin D3 to active vitamin D, can be stimulated by the vagus nerve.

Stimulation of the vagus nerve often results in the release of the **Vasoactive Intestinal Peptide (VIP)**, which is often at reduced rate in people with mold conditions.

NPY prevents some of the progression of the vagus nerve. NPY is an anti-anxiety and hunger-increasing hormone that prevents vagal stimulation from reducing the heart rate.

By regulating certain hormones, vagus nerve activation may decrease pain and anxiety and promote intestinal and cardiac health.

TAKEAWAY

The vagus of your nervous system plays a central role in relaxation and digesting. Optimum function of the vagus nerves promotes feeding, metabolism, mental health and intelligence.

Innumerable medical conditions such as IBS, leaky gut, IBD, GERD, brain fog, anxiety and depression may have vagal impairments. The vagus nerve stimulation is needed to work for digestive and metabolic hormones, sex hormones and growth factors.

Through yoga, meditation, prayer, cold weather, singing, fasting and massage you will naturally stimulate the vagus nerve.

Nutrients and nutrients that can improve the vagus nerve function include probiotics, protein, calcium, omega-3 and 5-HTP fatty acids.

Carbohydrate rich meals, ginger, and chili pepper, on the other hand, can suppress your vagus nerve.

HOW CAN WE MEASURE THE VAGUS NERVE PRODUCTIVITY?

The vagus nerve output is called vagal function or vagal tone. The strength of your vagal tone can be measured by the variability of the cardiac rate, directly linked to the regulatory system and your efficiency and health.

If a person has a low vagus activity or decreased vagus activity, the body has irregularities with the organ and digestive system controlled by the vagus nerve. If the brain cannot understand the data, the brain won't know how to solve any problems.

How does the immune system respond to the vagus nerve?

The initial immune system response is to inflame the irritated, wounded or contaminated region to protect the rest of your body. Inflammation is completely normal, provided that it is temporary. When your immune system has overcome the pressure, injury and disease, and it knows that your body is safe, your body begins to relax and stabilize again.

This is when the parasympathetic nervous system starts, which again is an important component of the vagus nerve. Injury stress or infection reduces the heart and breathing rates, and inflammation begins to dissipate.

If this nervous system doesn't work properly, though, the heart and respiratory rate will stay high and inflammation can remain constant. This opens the door to problems with health. But chiropractic care can help here.

Why the balance of your nervous system is so important

To keep your vagus and your entire nervous system healthy. All other systems of your body, including your immune system, function properly with a healthy nervous system.

If your vagus nerve doesn't work properly, it can lead to a long list of chronically inflamed problem health conditions. These health conditions include the following:

- Infection susceptibility
- Acid Reflex
- Skin Conditions
- Chronic Blood Pressure
- Heart
- Arthritis
- Osteoporosis
- Diabetes

Since the brain, spinal cord and the spinal neurons are compromising the nervous system, a chiropractic adjustment may help your nervous system and the vagus' nervous function. This condition includes but is not restricted to: This helps your whole body to work better.

BONUS: CHAPTER 7:
POLYVAGAL THEORY IN
PRACTICE

Our biology is hard-working in keeping us out of danger. As most psychologists know, our autonomous nervous system (ANS) is the body's rapid reaction survival mechanism. The ANS operates two branches for brief review: the sympathetic one and the parasympathetic one. The sympathetic branch mobilizes us in the fight-or-flight response to protect against danger. The less well-understood parasympathetic branch is generally seen as a unitary system that helps us through our defensive levels and regain calmness.

Yet it's a little more difficult, like they say. The vagus nerve is composed of the parasympathetic process, which begins at the base of the skull and makes its way down to the abdomen. It is divided into two major pathways, which each have a distinct neurophysiological disorder. One direction, known as the ventral vagal, responds to safety signals and encourages a sense of concentration and preparation for social participation. The dorsal vagal route, in comparison, responds to life-threatening indications that shut us down, get bogged down and separate us from others. A disassociated customer has found refuge in a vagal dorsal state.

Importantly, these security and threat measures are known by us. The three elements of our autonomic nervous system— ventricular, sympathetic and backbone— act as our largely unconscious monitoring system and read subtle signals of safety or threat in the background. A researcher, Stephen Porges coined the term neuroception to describe how our ANS scans security and hazard indications without any help from our minds. When you enter a noisy and crowded party and find foreigners huddled together laughing, for example, you will unintentionally gather rejection indications. The nervous system bursts to motion in a micromoment, signaling you to turn around and leave the parties posthaste or perhaps directly to the buffet and fill a dish.

Just then, you see one of the guests break from the crowd and walk to you. She reaches out her hand and presents herself, revealing and embracing her eyes. Almost immediately your breath slows down, your heart rate falls, and your body is relaxing to Ah, I'm now safe. Your ANS has just led you to a sympathetic state which allows you to fully connect to what Porges calls your social commitment system. Now you're cool, ready to connect — and perhaps start a new conversation.

Polyvagal Informed Therapy

Regarding the polyvagal perspective, the therapy's main goal is to help clients find solutions for moving away from a dysregulated status–be it a bogged-out "dorsal vaguard" or hyper-aroused "sympathetic"–and returning to the biological safety and interconnection seat, "ventral vaguard." And as it is only possible to change our prevailing life story from a point of ventral vagal, both psychologist just client need to be able to accurately recognize their nervous systems at all times– both during the therapy session and across the globe. Only when people can remember their position on the multi-vaguard will they start their journey back to calm and connection.

Notice that I said that both therapist and client need to be aware of their autonomy. Emotional healings can only be done when a clinician and client builds a trustworthy connection between the nervous system and the nervous system. Unconsciously, clients constantly receive subtle signals from their counselor through speech, eye contact, body posture and expression of the eyes, from a subtly wrinkled brow to a certain gesture of the hand. During the session, customers respond constantly to these signals through sympathetic activation, dorsal shutdown or ventral openness and trust. From a flexible viewpoint, healing relationships between client and counselor also allow therapists to know their own ANS and to learn how to manage this in the middle of any session.

Knowing your Nervous System

Today, most people are treated with a general understanding of the concept of "body-mind," the notion that their physical and emotional nature works in conjunction with each other. Nevertheless, I found that relatively few people understand the precise way in which the body produces emotional experience which in turn leads people to behave in predictable ways which create and maintain a story concerning themselves and the world in which they live. I help customers create a clear map of their own autonomous nervous systems, so they know how to react to ease and distress.

Brain chemistry can be like picturing a storm. Although we can imagine bad weather, it's hard to imagine that weather will change. Nevertheless, the polyvagal based concept of Stephen Porges provides a useful image of the nervous system that can direct our efforts to assist our clients.

Porges ' polyvagal idea originated from his vagus nerve experiments. The vagus nerve represents the para-sympathetic nervous system, the soothing part of our mechanical nervous system. The para-sympathetic component of the autonomous nervous system matches the sympathetic active portion of the nervous system.

Three - Part Nervous System

Our nervous system was presented as a two-part antagonistic system before the polyvagal theory with less calming and more soothing signals and less activation. Polyvagal theory identifies a third kind of reaction of the nervous system called the social engagement system by Porges, a playful blend of activation and calming based on the unique nervous influence.

The system of social interaction allows us to establish relationships. Helping our consumers use their public participation system to make their coping strategies more flexible.

The other two elements of our nervous system help us handle life risks. The two responses induced by these two parts of the nervous system are already established by most of the counselors: a sympathetic fight or flight and a parasympathetic shutdown which is sometimes referred to as freeze or faint. On the other hand, the use of our social commitment system requires a sense of security.

Polyvagal theory assists us in understanding that the two branches of the vagus nerve relax the body. The dorsal branch of the vagus nerve is stopped or freezing or fainting. This reaction will sound like the tired muscles and lightness of a bad influenza. It can shift us in immobility or dissociation when the dorsal vagal nerve closes the body. The dorsal branch controls the portion of the body below the diaphragm and also affects the heart and lungs.

The ventral branch of the vagal nerve controls the movement of the body over the diaphragm. This is the division that represents the system of social engagement. The ventric vagus nerve dampens the frequently active state of the skin. Picture of a horse controlling you back to the stable. You should pull on and release your kidneys in complex ways in order to ensure that the horse holds pace. The ventral vagal nerve also permits complex activation, thereby providing a qualitative difference than sympathetic activation.

Ventrally subtly released into operation takes milliseconds, while sympathetic activation takes seconds and includes different chemical reactions which are like losing the rings of the horse. Furthermore, once chemical reactions to the fight or flight have begun, it takes our bodies 10-20 minutes to get back to our pre-fight / pre-flight situation. Such kinds of chemical reactions do not include core vagal releases into operation. We can thus make faster changes between stimulation and relaxation as we can when we monitor the horse using the kidneys.

You will see some dogs who are scared if you go to a dog park. They display combat or flight behavior. Some dogs are going to show a play wish. This message also takes the form of the downside dog pose that we humans have hijacked in yoga. If a dog gives this warning, it leads to an extreme level of excitement. This playful energy, however, has a very different spirit than the intensity of combat or flight behavior. This funny nature characterizes the system of social engagement. If we feel that our world is secure, we function through our social engagement framework.

Trauma's Effect on Nervous System Reaction

If we have an unresolved injury, we will live in a constant fight and/or flight version. We might channel this fight or flight fear into tasks like house cleaning, leaves packing or working at the fitness center, but such things will have the same feeling as if they had been done with a biological approach to social interaction (think "Whistle While You Work").

No activity successfully channels their fight-or-flight sensations for some trauma survivors. As a result, they feel trapped and shut down their bodies. Such customers that live in a perpetual shutdown version.

Peter Levine, Porges ' lifelong friend and colleague, has researched shutdown response by watching pets and interacting with clients. In Waking the Tiger: Healing injury, he describes that a shudder or shake from the shutdown requires suspended battle or air power to unload. We will wake up in a life-threatening situation if we have a shutdown and a chance of successful survival. As consultants, we must understand this change from shutdown to fight or flight in the move from a customer to anxiety.

But how do we help our consumers step into their biology of social commitment? When consumers live more dissociatively, depressedly, shut down, we need to temporarily help them move into battle and flight. When customers experience battle or flight speed, we need to give them a sense of safety. If you can feel safe, you can switch to your social engagement process.

Clients may take dissociatively shutdown responses by implementing more concrete body-awareness strategies, which are part of Cognitive Behavioral Therapy and Dialectical Behavior Therapy. When customers are more in their bodies and more able to cope with momentary muscle tension, they will wake up from a shutdown reaction. When customers switch from shutdown to flight sensations, the rethinking strategies, which also belong to CBT and DBT, will advise customers to assess their security more accurately. Reflective listening strategies may help customers to feel connected to their consultants. It helps these clients to feel safe enough to become biological for social participation.

Specific Aspect of Vagal Nerve Functioning

Porges has chosen the name Social Engagement System as the ventric vagal nerve affects the mid ear, which blocks out background noises to make hearing the human voice easier. It also affects the ability to render communicative facial expressions. Eventually, this affects the larynx and therefore the vocal tone and vocal mode, which allows people to create sounds that relieve one another.

In 2011, Porges has explored the use of sound stimulation to train mid-ear muscles since publishing The Polyvagal Theory: Neurophysiological foundations of feelings, attachment, interaction, and self-regulation. Clients with a malfunctioning social engagement mechanism may have inner ear problems that make it difficult to obtain comfort from the voices of others. As experts, we are mindful of our speech habits and facial expressions and curious about the effect these things have on our clients.

Based on his understanding of the actions of the vagus nerve, Porges states that the para-sympathetic nervous system is triggered by exhales longer than inhales for a period of time. Porges was a clarinet player in his youth and remembers the instrument's influence from breath patterns.

As a dance instructor, I know that extending exhalations helps customers who have a feeling of safety in the midst of battle or flight response. I have found that conscious breathing can activate the fight-or-flight response for clients who remain in some sort of shutdown. When this occurs, the fighting or flight energy must be discharged by movement in order to ensure customers have a sense of security. Of example, these customers may need to run or hit a pillow. Such therapeutic strategies are explained by the structure of defense system working.

Respiratory sinus arrhythmias are a strong ventricular index. This means that we now have tools to research the effects of body therapy and expressive treatments.

Polyvagic theory in my practice

The following is an example of how I used polyvagic theory with a patient who had medical trauma while she was born.

The client whom I saw some time ago mentioned how sleepy and admitted that it was difficult to reach our session this day. Your doctor recommended Zoloft to treat anxiety induced by the birth of her first daughter. The customer and I had processed their depression as a stressful reaction before.

This patient attempted suicide during the years before he came to see me and contributed to medical procedures that added to his distress. Through our research, she understands that the anxiety she feels when it comes to emotional reactions in confined circumstances. She's lived much of her life in constant combat-or-flight response mode.

On that day she was relieved of being less anxious, but she dreaded the exhaustion that followed Zoloft's assistance in soothing her feelings of battle or flight. I saw this tiredness fear as a fear of vagal dorsal shutdown. We addressed the possibility of a new form of activation from this tiredness. I asked if she wanted to do some expressive art that would make gentle, expressive movement possible. She shuddered and called her preference for less subjective things.

We spoke of the presence of some sort of life that is still free. We talked about the possibility of being in a fun position where only choice is not right and wrong. We remembered that she and her family had worried since her birth that her health would fail again. The culture in which she grew up facilitated the operation of the nervous system intended for life-threatening conditions. I suggested that Zoloft would try some more relaxed and playful kinds of subjective experiences when it calmed their fighting or flight activation.

"It feels like you're trying to create another me," she responded. I knew it might sound like I figured she might be someone she wasn't. Yet I clarified that the idea that she could be herself in a different way was what I meant.

The client told me that she had a new grandparent's book with a section on playing. She said she'd say she'd read it. At the same time, she said that she could not and could not handle the Zoloft. Nonetheless, she was introduced to and experimented for a moment or two with the idea of this new, more playful way of being.

Getting the picture

As therapists armed with numerous theories, we should represent the structure of the defense mechanism. We can see transitions from battle to shut-down when customers are stuck. We can also understand the transition from shutdown to battle or flight, which can turn into a biology for social interaction if and when the customer is certain.

Most consultants will probably recognize fight-or-flight and shutdown activities before the concept of polyvagus. You will probably sense a distinction between life-threatening security responses and responses that represent what Porges calls the social engagement process. Polyvagal theory intensifies this understanding by recognizing that playful anticipation and restaurant surrender have a special impact upon the nervous system.

Many consultants understand brain science, but find it difficult to envision how the data is used. Thanks to the polyvagal theory, we now have an overview of the function of the ventral branch of the vagus nerve.

CONCLUSION

The Vagus nerve could be regarded as a super highway between your body and brain-we talk a lot about the link in yoga! The messages fly along its five paths, with four routes that provide information from the body to the brain and one path that moves data from the brain to the body. This is the most obvious physical representation of the relation between mind and body. The Vagus nerve also detects and influences the inner world (through its sensory neurons) (through its motor neurons). Because much of the work of the nerve depends on how the information goes, from here on we can divide the information into body-to-brain and brain-to-body.

Some of Vagus ' functions have been known for a long time, while others have been discovered recently. Without doubt that in the coming decades, we will continue to learn ever more, as electrical stimulation of the Vagus nerve is becoming an alternative to treatment under conditions such as autism, rheumatoid arthritis, and depression.